My
FITNESS
EXPERIMENTS

VC CHOWDARY

Printed in the United States of America
ISBN: Softcover   978-1-63871-849-9
           eBook   978-1-63871-850-5
Republished by: PageTurner Press and Media LLC
Publication Date: 01/06/2022

To order copies of this book, contact:
PageTurner Press and Media
Phone: 1-888-447-9651
info@pageturner.us
www.pageturner.us

My
FITNESS
Experiments

by
V C Chowdary

To

My *Mother*, who moulded my Personality with her Humility, Kindliness and Generosity,

My *Brother*, who has been the inspiration behind my Perseverance, Faith and Confidence,

My *Father-in-law*, who continues to be my role model for Health, Fitness and Propriety,

Acknowledgement:

Thank you, Oxford University Press for teaching me English through your Oxford Advanced Learners' Dictionary.

Thank you, Microsoft for enabling me to write and repeatedly rewrite with ease in your Microsoft Office 'Word'.

Thank you BlackBerry for facilitating me initially to write (different parts of the book while travelling or while I was in my farm) and conveniently send it to my mail box.

Thank you, Google for helping me search for information on anything.

Thank you, Wikipedia for giving me innumerable articles and knowledge on different topics.

Thank you, YouTube for showing me several talks on health and fitness.

Thank you, Dictionary.com for enabling the use of dictionary so un-laborious.

Thank you Page Turner for coming forward to publish my book. I thank Mark Alvarez, Rissa Saberon, Anton Belleza and the entire team of Page Turner for their help.

I thank my childhood friend Mr. P. Gopal Reddy, who has painted my own exercise images for the book. We were doing home work (school projects) together as children too. I used to write and Gopal used to draw.

I acknowledge the help of my medico children, son Shashanka and foster son Shreyas who read the manuscript and helped me in correcting and in making the improvements to the content.

Contents

Prologue

The driving force of any civilization is sharing and passing down of knowledge and experience from person to person and from generation to generation. The sharing and passing down help to prevent old mistakes and avoid reinvention of the wheel. It also helps to develop further on the existing knowledge. Such improvements over generations in different fields of knowledge have driven all the progress and development in the world. The sharing and passing down of knowledge and experience became easy and effective with developments in language, writing, printing, radio and television and information technology. The institutionalization of knowledge dissemination in the form of education was a major milestone in civilization.

It is well known that the societies of the modern world who have proper systems of recording, imparting and passing down knowledge have progressed better. Therefore anyone who acquires any knowledge should record and pass on to others. Such knowledge whether one benefitted from it or not, will be useful to others because people get to know what works and what does not. This recounting of my experience and experiments in fitness and health is one small contribution by a non-professional to the vast knowledge base in the field.

My over four decades of experiments in fitness and health helped me to be what I am today - an active, healthy and happy man. Starting in my late teens, I tried many ways, things and means to keep myself fit and healthy. The attempts were half hearted initially. But progressively my efforts became very serious and sincere. They varied from simple walking and swimming to complex gym-exercises and even devices such as Bullworker (a pull and press device) and vibratory belts. I tried several other systems too. I practiced *yoga* and did '*Pranayamam*'. I enrolled myself in The Art of Living Foundation's Basic Course, aptly called 'Happiness Program'. I also attended a 10 day *Vipassana* Meditation Course conducted by the Vipassana Meditation and Research Centre (absolutely free of charge! no course fee, free food and free accommodation. It costs nothing to learn such an invaluable practice that helps to be cool, happy and healthy!) I have tried different diets over several years and now arrived at a healthy and balanced diet. Though my experimentation and further improvements continue, I have now come to a stage where I can say I am comfortable with my fitness level and am confident that I can maintain it. I neither have a six-pack abdomen nor aim to have one. But I do have a healthy and able body which is fit enough for my age.

Though I am careful and keep consulting doctors for any health issues that I face, I have never sought any professional help for fitness. I also don't depend on medical experts for advice on prevention of health problems. But I discuss with anybody who has some knowledge or interest in the subject. I have read and gained knowledge from sources such as fitness books, health books, newspapers, periodicals and internet. More than that, decades of my continuous focus on the issue has helped me to gain a measure of insight and full confidence. I am confident that my experience will, at least to some extent help, you the reader, in planning and reaching your fitness and health goals.

What follows is an account of why, what and how of fitness and health of a layman by a layman for the layman. It is an autobiographical account of my journey to fitness and good health in Part-I to Part-V. Part-VI is preparation for my life ahead. The exercises I do and *Yogasanams* I practice and benefits are also explained in Part-VI. My pictures of walking and Yogasanaams are given near respective explanation for a better understanding of how they are done.

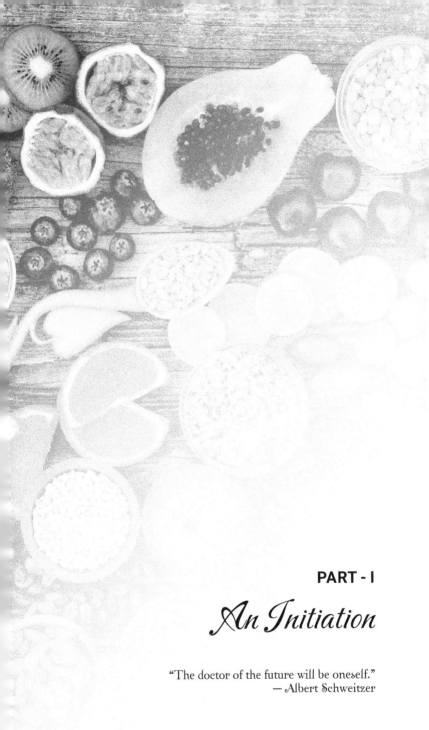

PART - I

An Initiation

"The doctor of the future will be oneself."
— Albert Schweitzer

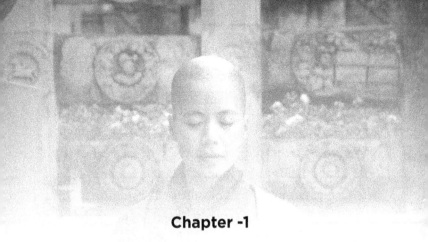

Chapter -1

This Is How It Started

"Why don't you run a few rounds of your college ground every morning? Running will help you to boost your body's resistance power", said the friendly doctor. "That is the best way for you to prevent your frequent bouts of colds and throat infections" he said. My efforts to be fit and healthy and my fitness experiments started with the advice of this kind doctor at my hostel's part-time clinic. Since my joining in the college a few months before, I hardly had any physical activity. My hostel was within the college campus and I didn't play nor knew how to play any outdoor games. It then dawned on me that this problem of frequent colds and infections was not there when I was walking or cycling to my high school. My lack of physical activity, I reasoned and realized, was responsible for my low disease resistance.

I was frequently sick as a child too. A posthumous child, born a month after my father's death, I was very precious to my mother. My brother, two sisters and cousins, who were all much older, were over protective of their kid brother. Effectively, I was raised as an only child of the family. Brilliant by the standards of single-room, solo-teacher and all of thirty students' elementary school and being the youngest member of a respected big-farmer family, I was cynosure of all eyes. But all the attention and overprotective care deprived me of the fun and frolic of chasing calves, handling bullocks, playing leapfrog and roaming in the fields. While all other boys of my age were trying their hand for fun at a plough in the field or learning to drive a bullock-cart, I was scared to be anywhere near those activities. I wasn't allowed to mix much with other children of the village for fear of falling into wrong company of naughty-boy gang. The restrictions conveniently suited my weak body and docile temperament.

Many of the children, raised by rustic and illiterate parents, were so much distracted with their playing and outdoor adventures that they would hate to attend school. The teacher would send a team of strong boys to track the truants and forcibly bring them, even against the wishes of the parents, to school. In spite of such care by the teacher and despite the Government giving free education and free books to every child regardless of class, creed and income of parents, dropping out of school was the norm of the day. Most of the children would stop attending school after Standard II or III (Second or Third Grade). Girls, if at all enrolled in school, were invariably made to drop out of school by their parents at age seven or eight, as though it was a sin to continue any more. I was, in fact, the only student of the class in my Standard IV and V! (Grade Four and Grade Five)

Most of my time was spent around my home and that of my paternal aunt near our home, which was simply called 'that house'. Even with the limited movements between those two houses, 'that house' and 'this house' I was a walking disaster. I would often fall and injure my toes, knees and forehead. And with half a dozen resident farm hands and scores of other workers at our family's disposal there was no work that I could contribute at home or in the farm. I would not be allowed to learn or try any of the 'manly' household chores like drawing water from the well, splitting firewood logs, milking, feeding and watering the cows or sweeping the cattle shed. If I wished to visit the farm, I was allowed only occasionally under the care and supervision of one of the senior farm hands, who were all like members of my family.

One more habit that contributed to my dull and no-physical-activity life was reading. My maternal uncle had presented me with two interesting old *Telugu* story books. After reading those books I just got in to the habit. I enjoyed reading. Even in the evenings and before bed time I would read under the light of a kerosene lamp. Moreover, it was 'cool' to be a regular reader. A book in my hands, like an ornament, would make me someone special among the illiterate rural folk! My teacher also was proud of his 'studious' pupil and used to be pleased at my borrowing from the small unused wooden-trunk of books called 'school library'. By the time I was ten I had read all the illustrated children's editions of *The Mahabharatam, The Ramayanam, The Panchathantram* and several other story books in the old trunk.

While all work and no play made Jack a dull boy, no work and no play made me a sick boy. Sick I was all the time with a forever-running nose, cough and frequent fevers. I was a regular visitor to my 'family physician', actually a glorified hospital assistant practicing as a doctor with an official Registered Medical Practitioner (RMP) License in the nearby town. My doctor used to be very liberal with his penicillin and other shots on my behind, the only fleshy part of my sickly thin frame for the intra-muscular injections.

Every time I fell sick, the first thing my mother made me to go through, before going to the doctor was the 'red chilli' ritual to overcome the effect of an 'evil eye' that was supposed to have fallen on me. A servant would go to fetch the witch doctor, an old woman who was believed to be good at warding off malevolent influences. I would solemnly sit at the main threshold of the house. The witch doctor would hold a fistful of red chilli and salt in her left hand. She would then spit out and rotate her left fist in an anti clock direction repeatedly touching my forehead and the ground below. Throwing of the ritual salt and chilli into an open fire would end the ritual. The noise made by the crackling salt and the pungent fumes of burnt chilli meant that the malevolent influence had gone away!

Though it appears to me now as a silly and superstitious practice, I could never forget the seriousness and sincerity with which it was done. My mother and the witch doctor as well as all the people at that time believed that such rituals had beneficial effect. For all her time and trouble the witch doctor would be satisfied with a simple 'fee' of a betel leaf and a few betel nuts!

My high school admission in to Standard VI (Sixth Grade) changed my life drastically. The school in the neighbourhood town was three miles away from my village home. I had to walk or go on a bicycle to school daily with school bag as well as a lunch carrier. It was more often walking than cycling because mine was the only bicycle in the village of a hundred households. It was borrowed by anybody who had an 'urgent' work, at any time of the day or night. The bicycle was in fact treated like a common property of the whole village. The way mythical *Atlas* was condemned to bear the weight of The Heavens my '*Atlas*' brand bicycle was cursed to carry the weight of the whole village. The bicycle, made for riding on proper roads, could not just withstand the rough ride by simple rustics in bullock-cart ruts in the country-side. Almost every borrowing resulted in a breakdown and took more than a week's time to repair because my people had to give mind and time to carry it on a bullock-cart to a bicycle mechanic in the town.

My high school admission was a transition from the thirty student elementary school to a thousand student high school. It was also a shift from a one room school to a large campus that had many buildings and several playgrounds. It was a change from an affable single teacher to scores of indifferent or condescending teachers. A change of status from being a sacred cow in the elementary school to that of an ill-treated country cousin; disdainfully talked down to by seniors and lowly clerks.

There were seven sections, A to G in my Standard VI (Sixth Grade). None of the teachers knew the students by their names. Nobody cared about anybody. Each school bell would plunge the whole school into chaos and I would get lost amid the pandemonium. It was both disappointing and heartening for me. Disappointing because I wasn't getting the special treatment I had got used to. There was nobody to hover around and shield me. I had to get toughened and get used to the bullying of rough boys of the town. It was heartening because I wasn't watched over. There was also freedom to run around and play. It was a new found freedom I started enjoying.

The folkways of villages and small towns were such that whoever wanted to be good at studies was not encouraged to participate in games and sports. The students who were good in athletics and games, being naturally self confident, were considered disobedient, arrogant and naughty. They would often absent themselves from classes and were by default treated as poor in academics. The schools had altogether a different set of parameters for the students. One has to be totally submissive to be called an obedient and disciplined student. Timidity was a virtue. Being confident was considered arrogant. A studious boy, even if dull, was classified as an intelligent student. And a sportsman was branded practically as a gangster. It was rare that someone from a village or a small town did well both in sports and academics.

Too Much Too Soon!

Once advised by my good doctor I started running, as soon as I recovered from the cold I was suffering from, every morning in the college ground. It felt good. My infections came down dramatically. It was a great feeling to be relieved of the nuisance of endless coughs, colds, breathlessness and the sick feeling. I realized what difference physical exercise could make to my body and my well being. More energy and stamina lead to improved self-confidence. I was elated that I had discovered something great and useful. It was all fun to be in the college ground every morning and it gave a great feeling. It was then that I promised to myself; my health is my first priority and I will be regular for my exercises to keep myself healthy, always!

But the initial success was short lived. The success prodded me to do more intensely. I was sick again very soon. It was a case of too much too soon. I would start again after recovering from illness.

The body needs time to get used to the new stress caused by exercise. Exercise beyond a level means reduced immune function and risk of general infections like cold, cough and throat infections and even fever. It may also cause injuries in joints or sprain of muscles.

What level of exercise is good level? What duration of exercise is optimum? Over a period I concluded then that my body could take no more than 30-40 minutes of moderate exercise at that time. If it was intense I needed some rest intervals. Even this duration came down if I stopped exercise for a few months. After such a stopping I had to build up a threshold afresh by progressively and slowly increasing the duration of daily exercise.

Another way to look at our exercise now is an estimate of overall activity known as PAL or physical activity level based on calories spent, for which a calorie calculation devise is necessary. A smart watch like Fitbit gives a fairly good estimation of the live or real time calorie expenditure. A PAL score is a ratio of your total daily expenditure to your body's daily minimum maintenance calorie requirement, otherwise called basic metabolic rate, BMR. A sedentary modern day worker has a PAL score of 1.6, an old style farmer in a developing country 2.1 and a professional athlete 2.5. It is good if we can manage minimum PAL of 1.8 with exercises and with efforts to be active the whole day.

Modern health experts are of the opinion that just one session of exercise a day is not sufficient for good health, especially for those who want to lose weight or keep their sugar and lipid profiles in acceptable range. They advise that we keep ourselves physically active throughout the day. My Fitbit smart watch has a provision to remind me to take a minimum of 250 steps for 14 consecutive hours of the day!

The intensity of exercise or the ability to withstand exercise varies depending on the capacity of the body. Some bodies are naturally well built or genetically well endowed. Further, the capacity depends on the musculature, stamina and strength built over a period with the life style of the individual, food habits and the exercise training. All this can be judged case by case only. The individual has to closely observe his own body, his own stamina, strength and endurance and decide about the present capacity and future needs.

I did not know any calculations about the intensity of exercise during the initial years of my exercise. I knew only to run a few rounds of the college ground at a moderate pace and learnt by trial and error to avoid over doing. But such learning will adversely affect your exercise schedule. It is best to be in limits and progress step by step.

One way of avoiding overdoing is to keep track of your heart rate (number of heart beats per minute) and ensure that it does not exceed 70-85% of your 'maximal heart rate' (MHR) during your workout. Your MHR is calculated by deducting your age from the number 220. For example, if you are a 45 year old, then your MHR is 175 (220-45=175) and your target heart rate range is 122-149. If you are a beginner, you have to start at target rate of 122 and increase progressively to 149. Heart rate of 150-175 would be peak range and has to be attempted only when you are quite comfortable exercising and in any case it is not advisable to be in peak range for long. But in the case of professional sports persons it may be different because their peak heart rate often exceeds the MHR.

Another even more appropriate assessment of exercise would be calculation of zone minutes based on resting heart rate (RHR) and heart rate reserve (HRR). RHR is your heart rate when you are sitting idle and in rest. Your HRR is the difference between your RHR and MHR. Based on these values your personal zone minutes are calculated in the following manner:

Below Zones = HRR x 0.39 and below + RHR

Fat Burn Zone = HRR x 0.40 to 0.59 + RHR

Cardio Zone = HRR x 0.60 to 0.84 + RHR

Peak Zone = HRR x 0.85 and above + RHR

Whether you are a beginner or experienced, it is very important not to straight away plunge into a high intensity workout or stop such exercise abruptly. You have to always begin with a 3-5 minute warm up and end with a cool down of same duration. Warming up is just light or moderate exercises that prepares your body for the workout and cooling down is similar exercise that brings your body to resting position after the workout.

Chapter - 2

What is Fitness?

During the next few years, I just managed to avoid the nuisance of colds and cough. But I wasn't actually anywhere near being fit. In fact, the very concept of fitness was unknown to me. The only meaning of the word 'fit' known to me at that time was that of clothes. The olden day tailors would stitch shirts, shorts and trousers on a rough measurement. They were made big enough so as not to allow the child to outgrow the clothes. Clothes made for a child would last till they are faded, frayed and finally torn beyond repair. Only a privileged few could afford clothes made by a modern tailor who took exact body measurements and accordingly stitched. Only such clothes were known as 'fit' clothes. Ready to wear clothes were unheard of.

Interestingly and paradoxically the word 'fit' was used for some decades to mean 'tight' in general sense. 'Fit' was used as an antonym for 'loose'. Compared with the old style loose garments the new 'fit' ones were relatively tight. Anything, for example a bottle cap that didn't fit because it was too small in size, was said to be 'fit'.

The other known meaning of 'fit', since I was studying zoology, was as in Charles Darwin's *The Origin of Species* and survival of the fittest. Darwin's theory meant it to be an adaptation or suitability to the environment in which the organism lived. For me it also meant that I should; 'When in Rome, do as the Romans do'.

I realized much later that I was often sick during my dull childhood and elementary school life as there was no physical activity. My six mile daily walk to high school and fun and frolicking at the school exercised my body and I was relatively fit and healthy all my high school years. The health problem resurfaced as soon as I joined in the college because there was again no physical activity and I was totally unfit.

What is fitness? Fitness for you as a layperson is: being healthy and active with lots of energy to perform your work enthusiastically, be able to reach home at the end of a busy work day and still have energy to take your dear one out. You don't go to bed enervated after a hectic day - you are normal and cheerful. You can run, if required, a mile easily; you may pant and puff but will not double over gasping. You have strength to carry a big suit case without a stoop. You should, without a second thought, be able to climb a few flights of stairs when there is a long queue at the elevator. You can bend down to pick up an object off the floor or reach up to take a book from the top of your shelf. You can also stretch and retrieve an article from the far end corner under your bed. If you can do all these activities of daily life comfortably, it implies that you have stamina, strength and flexibility - the core components of fitness.

As a fit and healthy individual you are confident with a cool mind, clear thinking and a relaxed demeanour. You are naturally optimistic. Even in the worst of circumstances, you would remain realistic but would never be pessimistic. You have a Positive Mental Attitude (PMA).

Fitness is also not getting affected by frequent infections and other illnesses. Being fit, you will look and be healthy and energetic. You do not look older than your age. On the other hand it is most likely that you will look much younger.

The primary objective of a fitness program for a layman is good health, enduring health and health that lasts till death. It is natural that you occasionally face exercise induced minor ailments like cold, cough and throat infection, fever, soreness of muscles and sprains. But beyond that, your program to achieve fitness should never negatively affect your health in any way. Excessive exercise is actually harmful to health. People who build a good stamina over a long period and continue to do intense and excessive exercise may look lithe with slim body. But they appear haggard with pale skin, tired eyes, sunken cheeks and weather beaten faces. They may be fit but do not seem to live very long.

My general observation of the life of olden day land owners, farmers and farm hands shows to convince me that excessive physical activity, just like inactivity, is not a positive factor in health and longevity.

A typical land owner did not take part in any high intensity physical work, moved around in vehicles and otherwise was physically less active. He had more food and tended to be obese. He had many health issues and did not live long.

A farmer, on the other hand, was involved in long hours of hard work, physically active the whole day and had good food. He did not suffer from any health problems, but did not seem to live long enough. A farm hand was more like a farmer except that he did not get as good a food as a farmer got. He also did not have any health problems, but grew old very soon and had a much shorter life span.

The healthy man with a long life span seemed to be a landowner-farmer. He had good food and was physically active the whole day. He was not fat but could be overweight. The difference in his activity was that he did not participate in long hours of hard physical work. He was present in the farm, would start the work and leave it for others to continue because he has other things to manage and look after. He would on and off join the work and contribute short periods of intense labor just to motivate the workers. He would also not hesitate to join and contribute a full day's hard labour once a while in case of shortage of hands. He rarely suffered from diseases and also lived very long. The formula for good health and longevity seems to be healthy food, physically active life throughout the day and bouts of strenuous physical activity with plenty of rest in-between.

What is the Right Duration of Exercise?

How much exercise is good for you? It is, as mentioned in the previous chapter, different for each individual. Even for the same individual it differs with time and level of fitness at that point of time. An ordinary man's heavy and long 'work out' may be a mere play for a sports person. A layman plays a few games of tennis or badminton for his exercise. But a professional tennis player plays for hours every day. For him exercise is totally different and of higher order. As time progresses you have to continuously assess and revise your exercise needs and levels. You need to progressively increase the exercise duration. It is like upping the ante. If you don't up the ante, your smartly adaptable body gets used to the routine and your benefits of exercise are minimized. On the other hand if you overdo it, you have trouble again. The progress has to be slow and steady. It is generally recommended by World Health Organization

(WHO) and many health professionals that one has to accumulate a minimum of 150 minutes of physical exercise per week. Once you are able to regularly reach that weekly accumulation, you can progress in terms of intensity of exercise or shift towards different types of exercise. I am now comfortably able to log a total of about 450 minutes per week of *yoga,* aerobic and strength training exercise.

It appears that the body learns to do any work, read exercise, very efficiently with experience. An efficiently performed work consumes lesser calories of energy than normal work. Efficiency in work places lesser demand on heart, lungs, circulatory system and other organs. An able bodied man who is not a blacksmith has to struggle for hours to do the same work that could easily be done by a skilled blacksmith.

The shifting of a bank safe from an old building to a new place was an enlightening and thought provoking experience for me. A gang of four experienced men were able to easily manoeuvre a heavy bank safe to a new building within an hour. The same work was given up by a team of a dozen well built farm workers when they failed to move the heavy safe even after repeated attempts. It is because the muscles specifically required for the trade are well developed in skilled persons. Such specialized growth of muscles takes place when the same job is done repeatedly over a sufficiently long period. That, I believe, is skill building.

But in the case of exercises, our objective is to burn more calories and build and tone different muscles. We need to cheat the body by not sticking to only one or two types of exercises. You should have several types of anaerobic, aerobic and stretching activities in your exercise repertoire. By frequently changing the exercises, we do not allow the body to get used to and become efficient and reduce the calorie spend. We also have to give a totally new challenge, like a two-three hour walk, to the body once in a while. Different types of workout will also build and tone more muscles better than one type of workout.

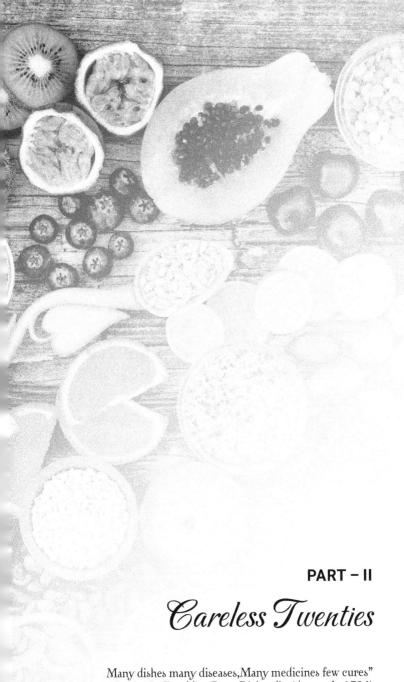

PART – II

Careless Twenties

Many dishes many diseases, Many medicines few cures"
—Benjamin Franklin (Poor Richard's Almanack, 1734)

Chapter - 3

Lifestyle Changes

My youth and good health coupled with my ignorance of fitness and health made me overconfident and careless during the next few years. My exercise regimen was very irregular. I would run a few minutes once a few days, do some push-ups and step-ups or pull-ups on the playground equipment, swing my arms few times and feel that I was doing great. I was so confident after 2-3 years of not so regular running and a few push-ups and pull-ups that I would try the Roman Rings at the university gym. It was fun swinging, doing dips and trying pull-ups on the Rings. But it was too advanced an exercise for me to sustain. I had to give up after a few days as my body could not withstand the stress and strain of an exercise meant for and done by gymnasts and professional athletes.

During the years in the University in my early twenties, I was fit and comfortable with whatever exercise that I did. I was active with a large circle of friends. I would take long and leisurely walks with a few friends in the beautifully green university campus. I used to spend my spare time mostly in the large university library reading variety of books from the bewildering range, while most of the fellow young men roamed around the dusty and crowded town teasing girls.

Though relatively thin during the first few years of my twenties, I began gaining weight soon after I started working. But I hardly realized I was getting overweight, unless occasionally teased by some friends poking at my slightly bulging tummy that I was 'prospering' well.

I had just commenced my career as a Bank Officer. Getting used to the new working life after a leisurely college life was stressful. Working as a junior manager in weakly managed, trade-union dominated state owned bank branches with unending flow of highly demanding customers was more so.

My work tied me to the office desk for long hours. Ambitious, sensitive and sincere to the core, I would work till late in the evening sipping several cups of sugary tea. I used to be fully involved in work and wouldn't digest any negative remark about my work from anybody - be it customers or peers or superiors. I was conscientious and was constantly driven by my ambition to do more and more. And it should be done well. It was a continuous struggle to keep up the 'efficient officer' image.

The other part of my life, though different was also hectic. I was popular among friends and relatives as a 'good guy'. I would regularly get invitations for dinners and parties and would in turn host similarly very often. Occasionally, though considered a taboo in my society, we would indulge in a few drinks too. I was a good eater and would always eat with gusto.

Back home at my village, members of my family would expect me to be present for every festival and all important occasions. Their love and affection expressed through the special treatment I got would make me visit my village as often as would my leave of absence from office permit. That was in spite of the trouble of travelling by bus or train for more than 24 hours each way.

My marriage and children further enlarged my circle and added to my list of social and family obligations. More visits to the homes of new relatives, visits by relatives, weddings to attend and above all managing a home and taking care of my family. This was all leading to two major changes in my life, in particular for my body. There was more and more of high calorie food and less and less of time for any exercise. It was also too trying and troublesome a task to balance my work and career, personal finances, family and social commitments. All these changes had trouble in store for me!

The effects of unhealthy food or lack of physical activity on the body are very slow, delayed, inconspicuous and rarely direct. If we eat contaminated food we may get sick very soon and realize that the food has caused the problem. But if we eat too much of calorie rich dessert day after day we never realize its negative effect immediately. The cause-effect relationship is not linked. We always tend to knowingly ignore the long term well being for a short term comfort and pleasure. Unhealthy eating as well as physically inactive life are both addictive in nature and are aptly classified as two of the seven sins, gluttony and sloth. We continue to enjoy unhealthy food and physically inactive life month after month and year after year, till we are initially diagnosed with one of the lifestyle diseases such as diabetes or hypertension or heart disease. From then on starts our association with doctors' clinics, diagnostic labs, pharmacies and hospitals!

Chapter - 4

Heartburn

By my mid twenties I was suffering from heart-burn and acid regurgitation. It needed regular medication. I would often chew antacid tablets or gulp down liquid antacids after every meal. My initial impression after consultation with my doctor was that my spicy food was the cause of my hyper acidity. He advised me to take only bland food. Changing food and even changing doctors did not help. I was frequently feeling uneasy waking up in the middle of the night with acid in my throat and burning in my chest and abdomen. I was quite sick and unfit.

Trying grandma remedies like milk or buttermilk were also not of any use. I even tried drinking more water as a way to dilute the acid in the stomach. It was giving only a temporary relief at best. It was making me uncomfortable too with frequent visits to the rest room. I learnt though that water plays a critical role in my overall health and well being by hydrating the body tissues, helping to remove waste from the body and keeping the skin healthy. But I found in the long run that it is not practicable to fix a particular quantity for consumption of water. The best way to drink the required quantity is by routinely observing the color of urine. It should be close to color of water. A color of pale straw should make you to drink more water. A shade darker beyond pale straw should alarm you and make you think.

Heartburn - not in any way connected with heart - is a burning sensation or in some cases even pain in the stomach and oesophagus due to hyper acidity. In this condition stomach produces more than necessary amounts of acid. The walls of the stomach, which are generally coated with a layer of mucous, get exposed to the acid when there is too much of it in the stomach sac.

The exposed walls of stomach or intestine if untreated will soon get 'eaten away' by the acid and cause soreness. The affected portion of the stomach or intestinal wall, over a period, may develop into a wound like condition called ulcer. An ulcer is very painful and causes stomach aches. It may cause severe bleeding and anemia too. An untreated ulcer could turn in to a life threatening perforation in the stomach wall; it causes multiple infections or damage of sensitive internal organs due to leakage of stomach fluids into the body cavity.

Hyper acidity also causes, in some cases, acid to push through the esophageal sphincter and reach up to throat. Medically known as Gastro Esophageal Reflux Disease - GERD, it is a flow of stomach contents back up to the throat in a spasm. It creates a very unpleasant burning sensation in the throat. It may cause, in addition to all the problems associated with hyperacidity, sore throat, cough, other lung infections and hiccups.

Though there are many reasons for getting the condition, my GERD would have been due nothing but to my overeating and my bad food habits. I enjoyed eating full. I would often deliberately skip breakfast so that I got very hungry and ate well till surfeited and sated. When the stomach is full of undigested food, the sphincter, a ring shaped muscle, which controls the movement of food between stomach and esophagus cannot maintain its grip on the contents. The over filled stomach pushes the acid mixed contents in to the esophagus and up to the throat.

In addition to excessive eating, obesity is also a major cause of GERD. Excessive visceral fat in the abdomen pushes up the contents of the stomach and causes acid reflux. Pregnancy and a medical condition called Scleroderma are also known to cause the problem. There are some factors like eating more, consuming some foods which are not suitable to the body (unique to each individual), alcohol, fatty and fried foods and smoking which can aggravate an already existing condition.

I did not take any other treatment for my GERD other than what I got for my hyper acidity. Once I became sane and sensible in eating, the problem disappeared.

I had to continue using antacid tablets and liquids on a regular basis. It was initially on a doctor's prescription. But I got so much used to my problem that I would buy stocks of those medicines and use them when needed.

It appeared to me that my body was matching the production of acid proportionately with my intake of antacids. The relief would never be total even with increased dosage. My 'burning' in the stomach was not severe enough to warrant serious attention and not slight enough to totally ignore. I had to live with it.

Another interesting observation I made with my antacid medicine was that it sometimes appeared to me to be the cause of my hyperacidity. If I stopped taking antacid for a day, it would give total relief. The relief would be temporary and would last a day or two only. I had to restart the medication invariably again.

There were two occasions when I suffered from stomach ache. I had an endoscopy done by a gastroenterologist. I was relieved that there was no ulcer. I was advised to manage acidity or still better prevent hyperacidity altogether. I was prescribed 'H2 blockers' which worked better than my regular antacids. I learnt that while the antacids neutralized the acid already produced, the new medicine prevented or reduced production of acid. I felt much better with the new prescription. In terms of other side effects also the new medicine was much better. It had no 'after taste' of the antacids.

When I was using antacid tablets and liquids, the after-taste and unpleasant feeling in the stomach used to be awful. I would not mind or notice the unpleasant after-taste when the suffering was more. But when it wasn't severe I would hate the awful taste. When there was a bigger problem on hand, the smaller irritants were not noticed or seemed bearable!

Since I wasn't completely cured of heart-burn and acid reflux I decided to study and gain knowledge about the problem myself and started reading regularly about the topic. I learnt from various books that spicy food, onions, garlic, preserved foods, salty foods, fried foods, oily foods, meat, fish, fasting, over eating, under eating, tea, coffee, tobacco, alcohol and many other foods and beverages could cause acidity. Even milk, said to be the best and safest of all foods could cause acidity. I came to know that each human body is unique and each body has some specific friends and foes among food stuffs. For example milk may be friendly to your stomach and you may be comfortable with it. The same milk may cause hyper acidity in my stomach.

And as I read, I began realizing that I had to know more about my own body first. I had to remember what

I ate and what my activity of that day was and note the intensity of my hyper acidity. I had to link the response of my body to the food taken. I had to observe the reaction of my body to the activities of the day. I had to relate the state of my mind of the day to my hyperacidity.

My first finding was that my spicy food was not giving me acidity. I learnt in fact later that spices in general boost immunity. It is advisable to regularly have spices as part of the meal. They add variety to your food. They are known to positively affect your metabolism by stimulating the cell activity. But it should be ensured that spices are not deep fried. Care should also be taken so that spice content does not go to the extent of causing an upset stomach.

I realized at last that my hurried way of life, stress and tension at work were clearly the major contributors of my hyperacidity. Teaching myself to keep cool and a deliberately cultivated come-what-may-I-would-do-whatever-only-I-could attitude helped me to reduce my stress. It also brought some more relief from my hyper acidity. It was only a partial relief. Not total.

I would learn slowly that avoiding very hot food or fried food, taking smaller bites or smaller morsels and masticating well before swallowing would help and would give more relief. I also realized that eating too much, not eating breakfast, having too many cups of tea or coffee, even an occasional alcoholic drink would cause hyperacidity. While trying many grandma remedies on health I found that coconut water and dishes made of green gram were two food items that would give me very good relief from hyperacidity.

When we swallow hot food or beverages habitually, it seems that the hot stuff gradually melts away the mucus layer of the alimentary canal thereby exposing the tissues of the walls to acid. The exposed stomach walls start 'burning' first. If uncorrected, burned portion of the stomach becomes an ulcer.

The food we take should be well chewed. Chewing helps to mix saliva with food and breaks the food down in to smaller pieces. The masticated food provides more surface area for the acid to work on and neutralizes the acid. Inadequately chewed food has lesser surface area. The acid produced works instead on the stomach walls or reaches up to the upper alimentary canal with 'acid regurgitation'. There are, as already mentioned, some foods that evoke production of more acid than required by my body. Everybody has a different reaction for each food item. Each individual and his or her body are uniquely created. Each one has to observe and conclude what are good for one self and what aren't. An important point I learnt after three decades of observation and study is that sugary foods and fried food cause acidity. All along I believed that tea and coffee also were contributors of my hyperacidity. But I feel now that coffee and tea by themselves are not the culprits. It is the sugar that is taken with them.

Even too much of non sugary starchy foods also seem to cause the problem. It appears to me that the stomach tends to produce acid based on the quantity of food that we take in rather than the type of food taken in. More food begets more acid. It does not seem to have a mechanism to judge whether we have taken in protein or carbohydrate. If there is no protein in the large quantum of food taken in, then the acid produced is excessive and the excess acid causes hyper acidity. That is the reason why it is always advisable to eat some protein with every meal and in any case in moderation. Another interesting revelation to me was that I was comfortable on the days when I ate food that was my family's day-to-day menu during my growing years. Was it a mere psychological comfort? I wasn't sure. I am still not. Or was it that my digestive system was designed during my biological formative years for that type of food?

The relief I got from the changes that I made to my food was very good. I almost stopped using medicines for hyper acidity. But the problem did not disappear altogether. It has become very clear to me now that in addition to all the factors that seemed to cause hyperacidity, there is one more reason which I ignored all along. Hyperacidity is an immediate reaction of my body to indicate to me that I am taking in more food than it can manage with. I notice now that if I eat more in a party after a week of restricted and simple food, I don't have any hyperacidity. But if my feasting gets too frequent the problem reappears. My body can manage only an occasional high calorie meal, not regular or frequent feasting.

It has to be remembered, however, that the contents of the stomach are supposed to be always acidic. Stomach acid is essential component of digestion process. The acidity also helps in killing any foreign organisms that are ingested. Stomach acid is not bad. It has to be managed by good living and eating habits.

Between my twentieth and thirtieth birthdays I had to relocate myself to ten places in as many years for my graduate study in college, master's degree in the university, job probationary period and job transfers. Though it was fun and exciting to move and live in different places across the country, it was also tough on my body to adjust to the varying climatic conditions, social life and food cultures. Being a very curious person and an adventurous gourmet I would try and relish every new food that I came across. And put my body to test!

I finally managed to be completely free from hyper acidity and acid refluxes with these changes in my life style and eating habits;

1. Moderation in eating.

2. Eating slowly with proper mastication.

3. Eating several times a day instead of a few big meals.

4. Hydration of my body by regularly drinking water.

5. Managing to be stress free and avoiding a hurried life.

6. Limiting or altogether avoiding very starchy, sugary, fried and excessively fermented foods and alcohol.

The very strengths I had acquired - patience, and ability to manage stress and be cool - would later become a disadvantage for me in my employment in the next two decades. I had to take a major career decision later on account of these strengths.

Chapter - 5

My Vision

It was while I was on an evening walk with two of my friends that I realized I had developed short-sightedness. My friends could read letters on a name board of an office at a short distance from where we were walking. I could not read. I went to an ophthalmologist the next day. I was told that I was myopic and had to start using spectacles.

In my early twenties, I was struggling to fit into my new job. Getting used to numbers, calculations and tallying of books of accounts was hard on my eyes, or I thought so! Though it was fashionable to sport glasses at that time, I felt it was very inconvenient and a nuisance. But I had to get used to it and continued to use for the next two decades.

But by the time I was in my forties, I was increasingly uncomfortable with lenses. An ophthalmologist examined and prescribed bifocals explaining that I have a slight far-sightedness also along with my old condition of short-sightedness. The remedy was worse. I realized that I was entirely comfortable without any glasses. I was able to read even the fine print in newspapers and could drive on national highways without glasses. It was surprising for the doctor too. It appeared that both my sight problems had disappeared.

The doctor explained that in some individuals a pre-existing short-sightedness corrects as well as gets corrected by far-sightedness that sets-in in the forties. They got corrected mutually. Hurray! I was free from eye-glasses! I did not use any glasses for more than two decades thereafter. Again the use of reading glasses became inevitable in my early sixties. I need to use reading glasses that are of lesser power than that most people of my age use.

Evolutionary biologists are of the opinion that the now ordinary habit of reading, though universally accepted as a useful tool in advancement of the human society, is quite unnatural to the human eyes. Short sightedness or myopia is of relatively of recent origin in human history. It was rare in the past and seems to have started appearing with reading habit. It was revealed in an old study in Denmark that the incidence of myopia was just 3% among farmers and unskilled workers. It was a higher at 12% among craftsmen like carpenters and highest among university students at 32%. The unskilled workers don't need to see or focus much closely in their work. Such necessity for focus is more among craftsmen. Students need to concentrate on printed small letters for long hours. It appears that we may face more and more of myopia as we advance towards higher levels of learning in knowledge based economies.

One positive outcome of recent studies indicates that the incidence of myopia is less among children who tend to play outdoors more often. It is not just in the interest of general health but also in the interest of eye health that children should play outdoors often.

Medical science does not accept the belief of some people that exercises help prevent problems of eye sight. There does not seem to be any research evidence to prove or disprove such belief. But my experience suggests that there might be some benefit to eyes with exercises. I exercise by blinking, rotating and shifting the focus of my eyes on far and near objects. I also gently press my eyes and surrounding parts with my palms and fingers. All these exercises are done during the rest periods in-between in aerobic or strength training exercises.

Dental Issues

Another problem I faced during my twenties was sensitivity and cavities in teeth. My saliva was acidic due to the hyperacidity and acid refluxes that I was suffering from. The acidic saliva would slowly erode the enamel coat on my teeth thereby exposing the inner sensitive layers. It would also, coupled with improper oral hygiene and bacterial activity, cause cavities in the teeth. I had to get the cavities of a few of my teeth sealed by a dentist with silver filling.

Brushing is the most basic maintenance activity of the body. It is not seriously done by us though it needs just 2-3 minutes of our focus to ensure cleaning of all corners of the oral cavity. It is necessary to brush twice daily, of which once should be before going to bed. Regular flossing is necessary too. Flossing is compulsory after eating meat because the nutrient rich meat gets struck between teeth and invites germs to multiply.

In fact, even a simple habit of washing the mouth with water every time after a meal or a snack would help you considerably in oral hygiene. I always go to a basin in the wash room to wash my mouth even if I am given a finger bowl in a restaurant.

We are all aware that improper oral hygiene decays teeth, infects gums and causes bad breath. It is also known to cause throat infections and pneumonia. But the latest medical research reports that oral hygiene is linked to your overall health, especially your cardiac health.

Evolutionary biologists believe that one of the most important causes of death before modern civilization was tooth decay. A decayed tooth leads to a cavity which can be a conduit for infection of sensitive tissues including the brain. Such infections could be fatal.

One important lesson I learnt after decades of close observation of food habits is that mastication of food and regularly eating food that needs a thorough mastication is crucial to good health. We may not be able to follow what Horace Fletcher, 'The Great Masticator' of America said about mastication. He said that each bite of food should be chewed 100 times before swallowing. He is also popularly known to have said, "Nature will castigate those who do not masticate." However, there are a host of benefits when you chew your food thoroughly:

- Your teeth would be in perfect health when you chew your food well. 'Use it or lose it' principle is truly applicable here.

- Mastication gives a good exercise to your jaws and facial muscles. Toned muscles give a firm support to the facial skin. A firm skin makes you healthier and younger looking.

- Proper chewing of food helps in feeling full with lesser quantity of food. The system has time to convey the message of food intake to the brain. Mastication is known to trigger release of hormones that cause satiety.

- Mastication indirectly helps you in weight control as you tend to eat less.

- Swallowing of food would be smooth. Your risk of choking is minimized.

- Digestion of food is easy as mastication breaks down food into smaller and digestible pieces. The smaller pieces of food are more effective in neutralizing acid in the stomach.

- Mastication is known to stimulate production of stomach acid and enzymes that help in digestion of food.

- Mastication releases nutrients from the food as cell walls of the food molecules are broken in the mastication process.

- A very painful episode the present day youth face is that of wisdom teeth and irregular teeth. Since most of the children eat processed soft food, their jaws are not subjected to the stress that the jaw bone needs for its development and further growth. The lack of stress results in a shorter jaw that cannot accommodate all the teeth to come. They get overcrowded. The late comer, wisdom tooth does not have sufficient space on the jaw to grow and erupt. This necessitates the services of an orthodontist and also oral surgery. Regular chewing of a natural food requiring mastication or even chewing on a gum during childhood could probably mitigate the problem.

- One surprising benefit of mastication which most of us don't know is getting rid of ear wax. Regular mastication helps to slowly move any excess ear wax towards exterior, where it dries and falls off, mostly when in sleep. People who regularly chew well don't need to use any of those potentially harmful ear buds.

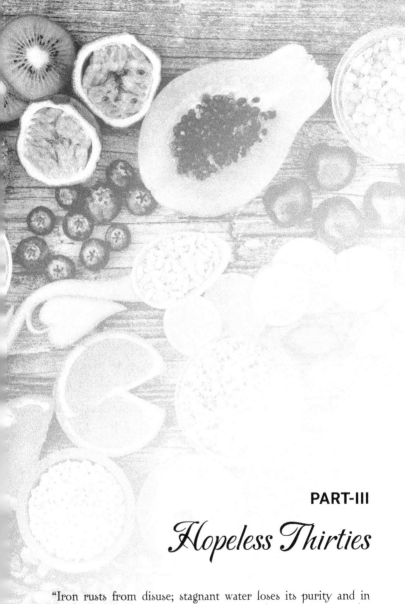

PART-III

Hopeless Thirties

"Iron rusts from disuse; stagnant water loses its purity and in cold weather becomes frozen; even so does inaction sap the vigor of the mind. So we must stretch ourselves to the very limits of human possibility. Anything less is a sin against both God and man."
—Leonardo da Vinci
(Inaction saps the vigor of the body too)

Chapter - 6

Unaccomplished Goals

While I was in the hope that my hyper acidity was manageable, I was not at all comfortable with my weight and fitness level. A healthy fit body with normal weight was my aspiration. Though life was comfortable and otherwise happy, these two major unattained goals were making me feel guilty and miserable. Guilty because I had made a promise to my-self long ago that I would exercise and keep myself healthy always. Though I wasn't suffering from any specific health problem, it was clear that I was moving in the wrong direction. It was logical and very likely that the life style dependent health problems that I wanted to prevent - diabetes, hypertension, cardiac problem and may be cancer too - could come knocking at my body any time very soon. My knowledge of health problems, which I acquired by reading regularly, made me more uncomfortable. The guilty feeling together with self forecast of my own health problems and resultant worry made my life miserable.

I also realized after many years of observation and thinking that exercising just enough or light exercise to keep common colds and minor infections away is like earning daily wages and managing expenses on a shoe string budget. A good exercise is like a good income that enables you to have sufficient savings too. A good amount of savings can help you to sail through rainy days also.

Some modern scientists are of the opinion that health and longevity of a person is primarily dependent on 'Organ Reserve'. Organ Reserve (OR) is the functional capacity of different organs to support and maintain vitality of the body. OR helps the body to withstand perturbations or sudden unexpected changes in the body and return to homeostasis or normalcy. It can in a way be equated with and corresponds to the skeletal muscle mass which again is proportional to your strength and stamina. The muscles also produce proteins and metabolites that are essential for recovery in times of illness, injury or exposure to toxins. A study supportive of this theory shows that the longest living among sports persons, who continue to be active even after retirement from their sport, are not marathoners or gymnasts but weight lifters. Weight lifters build big muscles and if the muscle mass is maintained thereafter by controlling sacropenia with regular physical activity they will have high OR capacity. A further study by European Society of Cardiology shows that muscle power is better than just muscle strength to reduce all-cause mortality. Power is an ability to generate force with speed, like when you get up quickly from a chair or climb stairs fast. We need to, on the other hand, generate just force when we push a car on the road!

When you are young, you have many times more OR capacity than it is required for the normal functioning of the body. As you age, the OR capacity comes down because of loss of muscle mass. You lose muscle mass with age primarily because of 'disuse' or not using of muscles. Reduced OR means inability of the body to withstand an illness or delay in recovery to normalcy. So, it is a simple rule of life that one has to use all muscles of the body by being physically active throughout, exercise regularly and build and maintain enough muscle to last long and healthy.

In a landmark tracking study of 20,000 men for eight years it was found that thin people who did not exercise had 200% more risk of dying when compared with obese men who had regular physical activity. More over the myth that health and longevity of a person is a gift from his parents and is largely dependent on his genes is belied by modern research. The latest estimations show that only 7% of your health is determined by your genes. The rest 93% is dependent on your lifestyle, mainly physical activity, healthy food and good state of mind.

Let me go back to my problem! My first problem was my weight which kept increasing continuously year by year. I was about to reach a Body Mass Index (BMI) level of 30 (More about BMI in the next part of this Chapter) and would soon graduate to 'obesity' stage from my 'overweight' status. My eating habits were uncontrollable. I was fond of sweets. Meat dishes were my favourite food. I liked to snack on sweets, cakes, biscuits and oily donuts in between meals. Sugary tea was almost an hourly necessity. Fruits, being health promoting, were readily available on the dining table tempting me at all times. I would also munch handful of raw or roasted nuts with morning tea.

My most favourite side dish was *Mirchi Bajji,* a type of fritter. Also a popular late afternoon snack, *Mirchi Bajji* is very hot and peppery. It is but a long chilli which is stuffed with spices, dipped in a thin batter of chick-pea flour and deep fried in vegetable oil. The snack is very high in calories but low in essential nutrients due to deep frying. The snack, if taken regularly, can also cause hyperacidity because it contains hot chilli and fried starch. Moreover food products such as *Mirchi Bajji* are generally bought from fast-food centers and hawkers where the frying oil is repeatedly reused. Such reuse can turn a healthy vegetable oil into a unhealthy trans-fat and also cause gradual buildup in the oil of harmful chemicals called 'polar compounds'. Polar compounds are proved to cause growth inhibition, organ enlargement and cancer in laboratory rats.

I was aware of my lack of control and I would often

decide and try to eat less. But if I willed myself to eat less during a meal, I would end up eating much more than the foregone food together with the next meal. Every food-stuff was tempting to me at any time of the day or night. I would often eat sweets and snacks made or meant for my little children. I was sure that I would fail the Marshmallow test even with both my hands tightly tied to the desk.

My focus during the second half of my twenties had been more on preventing hyper acidity. While I managed to eat slowly, started having regular breakfast and tried having regular meals, I was unable to control my portions. Whether it was breakfast or lunch or dinner I wouldn't be satisfied till I ate full.

The other problem was that I was very irregular for my exercise. I wouldn't even exercise on an average of one day a week. I was unable to exercise for reasons which appeared, to me then, beyond my control.

On the work front I was a senior manager independently managing a bank branch. It was a higher and more responsible role. Those were the days of manual accounting. Daily, weekly and monthly balancing of different books of accounts was a major time taking job. Added to that was an unending stream of MIS (Management Information System) Reports that were sought from us. It would take hours of regular time to make those reports.

Yet another reason for my time constraint was my how-best-I-could-help attitude towards any customer who came to me and asked for any assistance. Life was hectic and I was continuously occupied. I used to be so occupied with my work that I would routinely delay my lunch by an hour or even two. I wouldn't feel hungry or weak till I realized how late I was for lunch. Then suddenly I would be ravenously hungry and feel feverish. I wouldn't even have strength to get up or wash. But I would get normal within a minute or two of the first few bites of my lunch. Initially I was worried that it might be an indication of a serious problem. Getting tested for diabetes or any other problem gave a negative result. This irritant lasted till my forties and slowly disappeared without my ever realizing it.

The bank management wanted customers to have easy access to the managers. The arrangement in the bank was such that anyone can walk in to the manager's office at any time of the day without appointment. My office hours were just spent speaking to people; explaining, listening, clarifying, convincing, pleading, demanding, arguing, cajoling, coaxing, guiding and giving instructions. The consequence of this was that I could not do any paper work during the normal office hours. It had to be done sitting late after the office hours.

My family and social life was hectic too. I never wanted to miss any school events of my children. I was very keen to tell them bed time stories and also play quizzing games on *The Mahabharatam*, *The Ramayanam* and General Knowledge. My active participation and organizing was always expected by my family and extended family - be it a family get-together or a festival or a birthday party or shopping for a major family event - for I was an understanding, amenable and dependable member. I alone among the male members of my large extended family was counted upon to patiently wait, with a cash bag and credit cards in hand, when the ladies draped and tried every design, every color, every weave and every brand in the saree shop. The wait would be even longer at the jeweler's!

I was unable to have regular workout sessions, which I know now was more due to my lethargy and lack of determination than my busy work and family commitments. Having a guilty feeling nagging about my deteriorating fitness level did not make me any better. It was a helpless situation. I was continuously gaining knowledge and trying many easy options. I was also, as many lazy people do, looking for miracle solutions by experimenting with anything that I came across in pursuit of good health , fitness and weight reduction.

Body Mass Index:

The toughest part of a fitness and health program being body weight regulation, let's first learn about BMI before I reveal my failed experiments. BMI helps to know the level of being overweight or obese and also indirectly indicates fitness levels. Shedding body weight is tougher for people like me who have a propensity to gain weight. Body weight regulation depends more on determination, focus and constant awareness of one's own weight than anything else. An index like Body Mass Index (BMI), the current recognized standard of body weight and obesity is a useful tool to know the extent of weight in excess. BMI is also the most widely accepted indicator presently of fitness in terms of body weight. BMI is calculated by dividing weight in kilograms with square of height in meters.

BMI = Weight (kgs) / Height x Height (in mtrs)

BMI Range	Indication
<18.5	Under Weight
18.5-24.9	Normal Range
25-29.9	Over Weight
30-39.9	Obese
40 & above	Morbidly Obese

It is desirable to be in normal range. It is shown in many studies that having a BMI of 35 compared to a healthy BMI of 22 makes one 40 fold more prone to getting type 2 diabetes. There is correlation between higher BMI, 30 and above to several diseases including hypertension, heart disease and cancer too.

Being slightly overweight if otherwise fit is acceptable to many health experts. It is reasoned that fitness increases muscle and bone mass thereby making you a little overweight. Some research-reports also confirm, in fact, that other factors being equal, the chances of premature death are less in case of mildly overweight individuals when compared to the thin.

It is important to remember that not all naturally slim looking persons or those in normal BMI range are fit. To be fit one needs to have stamina, strength and flexibility too. If we recall the study mentioned in the previous chapter on 20,000 men, it shows that it is better to be obese and fit than thin and unfit. Dr. Robert Lustig . . . (More on Dr. Lustig in Chapter 13) is of the opinion that people who consume more sugar and high fructose corn syrup, which are added generously in processed foods and sodas, tend to be TOFI, thin outside – fat inside. Being TOFI is more dangerous than being obese, with fat spread all over the body.

A naturally slim person is at an advantage because he does not need to put special efforts for body weight regulation. Modern researchers are of the opinion that such slim people have an 'inefficient' metabolic system of energy usage in their bodies. For each of an activity of daily life (ADL) the body 'spends' more calories than required, thus burning away whatever eaten. On the opposite side the bodies of people with 'efficient' metabolic system of energy usage tend to save calories by using minimum energy for any activity. They spend less energy for each of ADL. The calories thus saved simply turn into fat.

The 'efficient' metabolic system might have been an advantage for the primitive man when he was struggling - hunting, foraging and digging - for his food. A food that was very low in calories. It is now a disadvantage for the modern man because of the abundantly available rich and concentrated food.

Chapter - 7

My Failed Experiments!

Exercise Bicycle

When I found that the maker of a popular brand of bicycles had designed an exercise bike, I was very keen to test and try. I was impressed the moment I saw it in the show room. It had both cycling and rowing operations and would exercise upper as well as lower body. I was very convinced of its usefulness and bought one very soon. But mere buying of exercise equipment would not exercise my body. I was too busy, or to be honest too lazy, to use it. I used it only occasionally. It remained at home as a show piece or worse, a stand to hang used clothes.

Exercising on exercise bike or regular bicycle is one of the best forms of cardiovascular exercise. In fact cycling is one of the few exercises where professionals experience the highest heart rates. Next to swimming, it is the most suitable exercise for overweight and obese people; because the body's bulk is borne by the bicycle seat. The knees and ankles are saved the trouble of bearing the body weight. The big muscles of the legs, knees and ankles are best exercised, at least initially, without the burden of the weight of the body. Once the body weight comes down and knees and ankles are strengthened, you can also do other forms of exercise.

Bullworker

A 'miracle' device that I came across in my efforts to be fit was Bullworker. Bullworker was advertised as a miracle exercise device that required just a few minutes a day to keep one fit and muscular. A very muscular and perfectly shaped body builder would appear in the mail order brochure to promote the devise and convince foolish fitness seekers like me. I felt as though it was an instrument designed for me and bought one without a second thought.

The device, a cylindrical contraption, worked like a piston. A cylinder like pipe fitting into another pipe of almost similar dimensions, it looked very promising. A spring inside would give a resistance and the required exercise to the arms and upper body. The workout was to shorten the device either by pressing the two ends of the device inwards or pulling out the thick opposing strings which connect the two ends.

It turned out to be a total disappointment as I did

not get any perceptible benefit out of its use. There were also some reports that exercises with Bullworker would result in shaky hands and that one would not even be able to hold a cup in hand without spilling the tea. It was a very convenient excuse for me to stop using the device. One important and valid negative point against Bullworker was that it did not exercise the lower body.

It has to be remembered that it is very important to exercise the lower body, mainly legs, as they are a large group of big muscles. These muscles place a very high demand on lungs, heart and vascular system, the exercise of which is of primary importance. It is essential to involve legs for cardiovascular exercise benefit. Leg muscles do not tire easily and can continuously make the indefatigable heart to pump and the lungs to oxygenate the blood. The continuous contraction of leg muscles pushes up the de-oxygenated blood back through the veins to the heart and lungs. It is for this reason that legs are called the 'second heart' of the body.

Acupressure Foot-Roller

Yet one more health seeking trial was Acupressure Foot Roller. It is a foot rest with several mildly sharp protrusions on a horizontally placed cylindrical roller that press the soles of your feet when you roll back and forth. It is believed to give the effect of acupuncture on the body. I used it at home, while reading the morning newspaper, for some time hoping that it would give some health benefits. Such benefits, if any at all, are neither perceptible nor proven. It may give some relief, mostly by way of diversion of attention, for some types of pain. All types of acupressure, without any doubt, are a type of simple massage. It may give some minute health benefits to the body by way of increased blood circulation to the massaged part. But it will not in any way give exercise to the body or help to reduce body weight.

Acupuncture, on the other hand, seems to work very well in pain relief, especially lower back pain. Though it is considered a pseudoscience by modern medicine, there are many who get relief from acupuncture treatment. Its explanation is given in Chapter 12 on Vipassana Meditation.

Lemon Juice and Honey

A grandma remedy or an alternative therapy suggested for overweight people was lemon juice with honey on an empty stomach. I tried that too. The therapy did nothing but aggravate my suffering from hyperacidity. Lemon juice has high content of citric acid. Adding an additional dose of acid to the already excessive acid in my stomach would naturally worsen the condition. I learnt the lesson the hard way!

But I found later to my amazement that there are some people who did get relief from hyper acidity by drinking diluted lemon juice mixed with a little honey every morning. One more proof that each human body is differently constituted!

Vibrator Belt and Body Fat

One more device I experimented with was an electrically operated vibratory belt. Again, I naively believed that it would melt my belly fat away just as the seller claimed. The seller claimed that the vibrator made the muscles burn fat by metabolically stimulating the muscle cells. The idea was very appealing to my gullible and receptive mind. It was one more example of my wishful thinking and a trial similar to that of a greedy get-rich-quick wealth seeker. I was also fooling myself to satisfy a part of me that I had tried everything.

Body fat is stubborn. There is no way you could reduce fat in a specific part of the body. It cannot be targeted. There will only be an overall reduction of fat if there is a general body weight reduction. If you want to reduce fat, you need patience, discipline and determination to fight it off in only a particular way, which is the hard way - reduction in calorie intake and exercise. My experience taught me that you cannot win a war on body fat or battle of the bulge unless you watch your food intake and at the same time exercise regularly. You need to necessarily invest time for exercises and also focus seriously on what you eat.

One deception that general fitness enthusiasts face is that of flattening of the abdomen within a few days after some types of exercises. When you do some exercises like sit-ups or some yoga postures the abdominal muscles get toned and pull the abdomen in. Initially it gives the impression that abdominal fat has disappeared. There will not be any change in body fat content or body weight. It just changes the body posture and gives an impression of a flat tummy. It may be good, but is not at all enough.

Fighting Fat - Strategy X Tactics

If you are an overweight person and intend to get fit, it has to be a war on your unfit and fat body. It is advisable to follow the Chinese General-Philosopher, Sun Tzu's important principle of war;

"Strategy without tactics is the slowest route to victory. Tactics without strategy is mere noise before defeat". Your program of regular exercise and moderate food intake is like a strategy and a slow route to your goals. If you join a health camp or a gym for a healthy weight reduction course, it becomes a tactic. Merely attending health camps will not help. It will only lead to frustration as you will fail. It has to be combined with your strategy. A tactic combined with your strategy is a sure, certain and reasonably quick route to success.

Coming back to vibratory belt, I learnt later that the US Federal Trade Commission had declared the ads of the sellers as deceiving several decades ago, in the year 1963 in their annual report. I also realized that most of the sellers also advise the user, though in fine print, to diet and exercise. I used the device for some time as massager and threw it away.

Body Fat and Inheritance

It is observed and recorded by researchers that adopted people whose biological parents were overweight tend to be overweight irrespective of the life style and eating habits of foster parents. On the other hand, children born to thin parents in Asia and Africa and raised in the high calorie environment of America also tend to be overweight. It is like heads I win, tails you lose situation. It appears that once you become overweight, your fattening genes get activated and pass down to the next generation in an activated state. All your descendents down the line tend to be overweight. Hence it is important that one ensures not getting overweight right from a young age not just in the interest of his or her own health but also that of future generations!

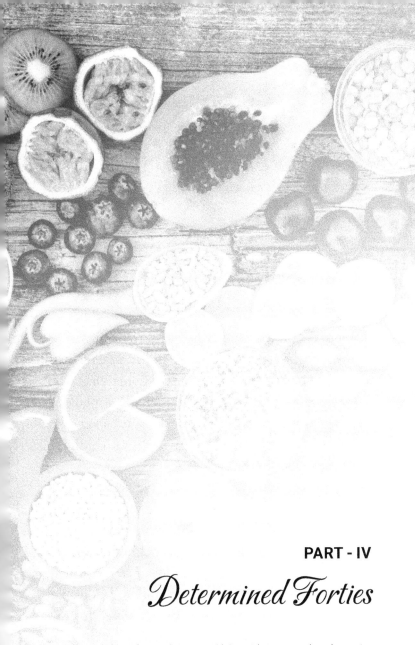

PART - IV

Determined Forties

"…ever did his duty in his way of life, with a strong hand, a quiet
tongue, and a gentle heart."
-Charles Dickens, Great Expectations (Pip's comment about his
sister's husband Joe, the blacksmith), Chapter 35

Chapter - 8

A Solid Resolution

For almost a decade I struggled to remain within overweight category. It was as if I had accepted my overweight body. My focus had shifted from trying to be fit to managing my overweight status-quo so that I didn't get obese. I was ashamed of myself. More than being ashamed, I was worried and scared. My fortieth birthday made me think, think seriously. A few years before that I had to attend on my brother who had undergone an open heart surgery. It was pathetic to be hospitalized and the hospital bills made us all feel worse. My personal finances were not in any great shape. Other than some agricultural land inherited from my ancestors, I had nothing else to be comfortable about. How bad would my life be if I were to suffer from a serious ailment? How about my family - All my dreams of giving the best education to my children and providing for a secure future for my family? It was very clear that for anything to be possible I had to be healthy and fit. I should be working and the working should be not for merely paying insurance and hospital bills.

My increasing weight, lack of stamina, total lack of body flexibility, advancing years and fear of onset of lifestyle diseases made me take a strong decision about my fitness. My transfer to another town was a starting point. It was an opportunity for me to start afresh. I was very determined to focus on fitness. The new determination to be fit was different from what was started casually and as a fun activity two decades ago. The new strong resolution was out of dire necessity. It was a desperate attempt to save my health and save myself.

I had already started gaining some knowledge about what was fitness and what was a healthy life style. It started with reading books and magazines on hyperacidity. I continued to read and concentrate on all articles about health and fitness. I started to notice that my favourite magazine then, *The Reader's Digest* carried monthly write ups and articles on health and fitness. There were some programs in the TV too, but it was never convenient to watch those programs because of my work or other occupations.

I started walking regularly - rain or shine, six days a week - at a moderate pace initially for about 45 minutes. The walking was progressively increased to 90 minutes a day. It was good till then. But when I started increasing the intensity of walking, I suffered exercise-stress induced minor infections like cold and sore throat a few times. But the recovery from those minor ailments was very swift. Every day I would reaffirm my commitment to the fitness goals I had set myself. To be effective I did the reaffirmation twice a day. Once in the morning as soon as I woke from sleep and again at the end of the day before going to bed. This helped me to sustain my efforts and be regular for exercise.

My strong determination would make me walk longer and with more intensity. Most of the days, I walked for nine to ten kilometers. It made me feel more confident. It was better than before, but sadly I continued to be overweight, almost fat. Fit but fat.

There is a school of thought that it is alright to be fit and fat. It may be better to be fit and fat than thin and unfit. But people who are fat, even if fit, suffer from many problems. The human body is designed for a certain weight. The knees, heels and feet cannot bear the burden of a heavy body. The cardiovascular system of the body cannot meet the demands of the large mass of the body. The heart cannot pump far enough in to the deep tissues. Many of the fat people, in spite of being fit, suffer from hypertension.

Let's get back to my story. Though I was very hopeful of reaching my goals, I realized soon that it wasn't easy. My first goal of improving fitness and increasing stamina appeared attainable and within reach. I was feeling much better than before. I wasn't getting exhausted even at the end of a very busy working day. In spite of being stout, there was a perceptible improvement in my body posture and general appearance too. But it was all relative. There was no mechanism readily available for me to assess my stamina or fitness. It was just that my position was comparatively better than before.

On the other hand I was totally disappointed with my weight goals. It was an easily measurable goal! I would regularly check my weight on a weighing scale. It was shocking to observe that my weight kept increasing slightly in the initial months. But my perseverance started showing a little progress after some time. But that wasn't much. I was not at all near my target.

One More Failed Experiment

My walking was getting monotonous. I knew that if I started getting friendly and began chatting with the other walkers in the park I would be wasting my time. I would also have to slow down once in a while just to allow the other person to catch up with me. That would work against my goal. So I started looking for another way to overcome monotony without affecting my exercise program. It was then that a friend suggested learning and playing tennis. He convinced me that it was the only game that was played regularly at the local officers club. It was a whole body exercise with good foot work, exercise for arms and several other body muscles. In fact some studies show that the longest living and healthy among players of different games are those who play tennis.

I bought a tennis racket immediately and joined the club. The coach asked me to practice by hitting the tennis ball against the wall. Though it was a little embarrassing to learn a new game like a child, I started 'wall practice' in earnest nevertheless. I reduced the time of my walking to compensate for the time spent for tennis. I also did brisk walking and some running to make up for the less intense 'wall practice'.

Within a few days of my tennis lessons I started getting severe elbow pain. It was expected because I had started something that was totally new to my body. I continued walking and running in spite of the elbow pain but stopped tennis. But very soon an aching knee and a tennis elbow took me to the orthopaedic surgeon. I was advised complete rest from all my exercises. It took almost a month for me to recover. The doctor also advised me to avoid walking on the surfaced hard roads. Thereafter I tried, wherever possible, walking on the sides avoiding concrete or bitumen roads. My efforts of almost a year, in terms of body weight, were wasted as I regained my previous weight during this one month rest.

I realized after a few trials that my arms were not strong enough to withstand tennis playing. It was probably repetitive hand movement for which I was not used to or incorrect playing, my elbow pain reappeared each time I resumed the game. I had to give up the game altogether and stopped my practice. Similarly I had to give up running too as my knees were unable to bear the running pressure of my overweight body. I did not attempt running for almost two decades thereafter.

Overdoing

My inability to bring down my weight to within normal BMI was making me very uneasy. I was certain that I was pushing myself to my limits with exercise. I had to be careful about exceeding the limit as it would be counterproductive. Overdoing would, in addition to soreness of muscles, inescapably stop my exercise schedule at least for a day, if not more. I observed that each level of overdoing would affect differently. If it was slightly more than normal, say I extended my walk by half an hour, it would cause disturbed sleep that night. I would wake quite early, after 2-3 hours of deep sleep. It would almost be impossible to sleep again the rest of the night. There wouldn't be mood or energy the next morning to go for my brisk walk.

The second stage of overdoing caused more damage. Higher intensity exercise, like when I tried increasing the time of my brisk walk or increased the number of repetitions or sets in my strength training, which I started later, would result in a cold or throat infection. It would take 3-5 days to recover. I would take a day more to resume my walks.

The third stage of overdoing, as I foolishly tested my limits trying to ape professionals once in a while, would cause a sprain and pain in any of the joints - ankle, knee, wrist, elbow or shoulder. That would take a week or even a fortnight to recover from. Moreover there was a possibility of cureless damage that could permanently impair my exercise schedule. So I had to be very careful about not exceeding the limits.

Some more known symptoms of over-training are: Increased heart rate, aggressive behaviour and depression, loss of concentration and other personality changes.

It appears that when you push yourself to the extreme limits of your body, you experience what is called 'over-training'. Over-training stimulates release of stress hormones to enable your body to repair damage caused to the muscles, tendons and ligaments. All the body's resources are diverted to the damage control job. That is when the body does not have enough strength to fight disease. Your immune system is weakened. You are susceptible to colds and vulnerable to other infections. The hormones may also affect the brain and cause different behavioural changes in different individuals.

When I suffered pain due to a little overdoing or an injury, the first thing a doctor did was to advise rest, often very long. But I learnt that resting should never be more than necessary. Resting too much is said to be counterproductive. Too much resting weakens the muscles that are rested. The body loses strength and flexibility. It can even reduce your balancing ability too.

Inflexible Body

I had got used to a routine way of life. Sleep in and get up from a two and a half feet high bed, sit in a revolving chair in the office - with quite a few assistants to move around and get things for me - turn left or right or reach for a file behind me without actually turning my body, sit in a sofa and watch TV or read, eat at the dining table sitting on a chair, do the routine morning brisk walk and feel that I was doing quite well with my body. But over a period of time the unused parts of the body as well as the routinely and repetitively used ones get stiffened, lose their original supple nature, become rigid and are not smoothly usable.

It happened when I was on a visit to my village for a festival. A relative invited me to have a meal at his home where there was no dining table. Everybody else was comfortable sitting cross-legged on the floor as is very common in India, especially for the meal of any religious festivals. I too used to eat sitting cross-legged on the floor during my childhood. But now it was a very uncomfortable experience for me and was amusing for others watching me sit and get up awkwardly. It was then that I felt the need for body flexibility. Fitness is incomplete or inadequate without flexibility. Flexibility is as important as strength or stamina or having normal body weight.

It is important to keep all parts of the body in proper shape. The body parts need to be strong as well as supple. I should be able to move, turn, bend, twist, curl and roll comfortably. I should, as mentioned in Chapter 2, also be able to reach up or bend down or stretch far with ease. I should, if necessary, look back and see behind while reversing my car. There should not be any stiffness in any part.

I took it very seriously to correct my stiff body. The first thing I did was to spread a mattress on the floor in my living room. The sofa set was meant only for the use by visitors. All my reading activity or watching TV was done sitting cross legged on the mattress on the floor. I also started to move around often at home and in office and get my own things and files. I bought a book on *Yoga* and started to practice some elementary *yoga asanams* or postures for improving the flexibility of my body.

Yoga

Yoga is much more than just *asanams* or postures for flexibility. But the discussion here is limited to asanams. Practicing *Yogasanams* would make the body very flexible and also help to keep one healthy physically and mentally due to general increase in breathing and blood circulation. The practice also helps in concentration and overall efficiency. But it cannot be a substitute for physical exercise. Yoga and physical exercise complement each other perfectly. While physical exercises contribute to the stamina and strength part of fitness, yoga contributes to the flexibility and good state of mind aspect of fitness.

But unfortunately some proponents and teachers of *yoga* make exaggerated claims to enlist people with assurance of cure of many ailments. The claims are based on the belief that the *rishis,* the sages of ancient India who designed or invented the yoga system lived long and lived healthy by practicing yoga. But such claims are not proven. Moreover the *rishis* of the ancient times walked miles of distances everyday even for food and water. They ate simple and raw food. They never ate calorie rich or processed foods. We have to remember that if a cure for one disease is prescribed as panacea for all diseases there will soon be more dissatisfied people than satisfied ones. Such exaggerated claims do not help to spread yoga.

Many yoga teachers include *Suryanamaskarams* or Sun Salutations as part of yoga. It is a desirable combination because *Suryanamaskarams* are similar to aerobic exercises. The *Suryanamaskarams* consist of twelve consecutive postures done in quick succession. These exercises are comparable to circuit exercises and give a good cardiovascular workout as well as flexibility to the body.

Dhyanam (meditation) and *Pranayamam* (breathing exercise) are packaged by default in *Yogasanams.* If you practice Yoga sincerely and correctly, you are also doing *Dhyanam* and *Pranayamam.* Each posture of Yoga involves breathing in and breathing out or holding breath for 8-10 seconds. Such breathing is Pranayamam. In the same way *Dhyanam* is practiced automatically as you continuously focus your mind on your breathing.

Fitness and Wealth – A Comparison

I realized during this determined-to-be-fit time of my life that it was quite hard to safe-guard whatever gains I had made in fitness and weight reduction. Even a short period of relaxation - not exercising or overindulging in food - would take me back to square one. Each time I went on a holiday or there was a wedding (series of several days of celebrations) in the family, I put on a few kilos of weight. I had to struggle again to reduce my weight as well as to rebuild my stamina.

The old adage says that health is wealth. Health as well as fitness are like wealth for one more reason too; difficult to acquire but easy to squander. Health and fitness acquired with determination and hard work of decades could easily be squandered in a short time. The best example for this would be that of 'Hand of God' Boy of Football. He attained great fitness, skills, fame and wealth by hard training and determination. He was a legendary figure with strong legs, excellent ball control and exceptional dribbling. He came to be considered as one of the most skilful players ever. But soon after retirement from active sport, he was suffering from morbid obesity, alcohol and drug abuse and cardiac problems. He was in financial trouble too with tax authorities after him. What he attained with great effort over a long period, he squandered very easily and quickly.

Two people with similar income and similar family size and working in the same office could be totally different in terms of their financial status. There could apparently be nothing much differentiating one from the other. One man is in debt trap and the other man is sound and safe with good bank balance. What differentiate them are the regular habits of saving: one goes by public transport and other uses a taxi. One plans well and buys things when they are cheap and other does on an impulse. Similarly health and fitness require several small positive activities that add up to achieve the desired result; walking a few blocks to office, taking the stairs instead of the elevator, active participation in every activity, cultivating simple food habits and the like.

Chapter - 9

My Food

It was becoming clearer to me each day that the only way I could achieve my goal of a healthy BMI was reducing my food intake. I also read several research reports that indicated that reduced food intake helped in good health and longevity. Termed as 'calorie restriction' (CR), restriction of food consumption was proved to prolong the life of laboratory animals. Rats which were given restricted food lived 40% longer. Can it be true, I thought, for humans too? Even my doubt that rats are not quite like humans for comparison was dispelled by an experiment on primates. In a research study by Wisconsin National Primate Research Centre, 76 monkeys (Indian macaque) were studied for over two decades. Half of the monkeys were allowed to eat *ad libitum* and the other half were allowed to eat 30% calories less than the control group's standard diet. The results of the study proved beyond doubt that unlimited food is quite anathematic to the body, its health and longevity.

Diet – Health – Longevity Study on Primates:

After 20 Years >	Survived Healthy	Survived Unhealthy	Total Survived
Ate *Ad libitum* (Control Group)	None	50%	50%
Ate restricted diet – 30% less calories (Experimental Group)	56%	24%	80%

While 50% of control group died during the study period, none of the surviving among them was healthy. Every surviving member of the control group had health issues. On the other hand, 80% of the experimental group survived. 70% of the surviving experimental group were free from any chronic disease. Another report on a study of post-war (WW-II) mortality rates in Oslo, Norway says that there was 30% reduction in mortality in Oslo due to restrictions in diet caused by food shortages during WW-II. Even the olden day wise sayings back home spoke of the stomach being only 'half full' for good health and longevity.

But all that knowledge and realization did not help me. It was difficult to take corrective action because of my weakness for food and habitual overeating. Human body is designed by evolution to overeat and store fat so that we survive famines and food shortages. Here I am in a safe, secure and shortages-free environment but my metabolism and instinctive behaviour continue to work the way they worked on my ancestors, hundreds of years ago. A few of my ingrained childhood eating habits also worked against me.

"Why do you eat so slow like a girl?" would be a gentle chiding in the village ethos. A boy was expected to eat well and eat fast. It was also - as nobody ate leftovers - a sin to leave food in the plate. In those days of poverty, famines and food shortages, when America was supplying broken maize under PL- 480 (Food for Peace) to mitigate hunger in the Third World, any excess food had to be given to the needy. And there was no electricity, leave alone a refrigerator to stock food. Food was cooked afresh for each meal.

My stubborn habit of not leaving food in the plate - based on the belief that 'food wasted was a sin committed' - would often make me eat more than I actually wanted to eat. It was in my control if I could serve myself. But if a host served me food, it was an embarrassing situation. It was customary for a host to serve food generously to the guest. I was accustomed to finish up all that was served in the plate!

My eating-fast habit also made me invariably eat more than necessary. The mechanism of my body to regulate eating, as explained in the later part of this Chapter does not seem to be perfect. The communication to the brain about eating is a chemical process. Several hormones, receptors and nerves regulate the eating and satiety process. The production of the hormones, their transport to the brain, their reaction and getting the feeling of satiety take time. By the time my brain received a message that I have had enough, I would have had had much more than enough.

When my repeated attempts to reduce food intake failed, I started to increase the bulk by eating more vegetables. It did help to reduce my rice and wheat consumption. But it did not make any difference to my weight. The calorific value of food we take is so high that even a small quantity is sufficient for the body. It appeared that the reduction in the intake I managed to achieve was of no consequence because even the reduced quantity was quite excessive for my body.

But when I tried eating a meal of more vegetables and fruits with minimum of other food I had to take an off from work with an upset stomach. My system could not process so much of veggie stuff. My stomach revolted and made me sick. It made me very weak too. I learnt later that crash dieting, just as I did with just vegetables and fruits, was actually counterproductive in my fitness program. Reducing weight by crash dieting results in loss of very valuable lean muscle. When the body is denied essential carbohydrates, proteins and fats it shifts into starvation mode. A body in starvation mode starts drawing the bare essentials from fat as well as muscle sources because survival is of primary concern.

We lose muscle mass also along with fat. When we regain the weight that is lost, the gain would only be in the form of fat. The net result is that in one cycle of weight loss by crash dieting we get back to original weight with more fat and less muscle.

A report by researchers at the Institute of Preventive Medicine (IPM) of Copenhagen University Hospital, Denmark drew a startling conclusion after a 30 yearlong study. They found that obese and overweight people who were trying to lose weight were at a 15% higher death risk than those who remained obese or overweight! This could be true because of the possibility that many of them might have tried to lose weight by crash dieting or any unhealthy means. Crash dieting or an unhealthy denial of nutrients progressively reduces muscle mass in the body. Reduced muscle mass means diminished organ reserve (OR). Diminished OR leads to inability of the body to recover from illness or injury or toxicity and results in higher risk of death.

One more potentially harmful situation the body faces when we crash diet is the toxic overload of muscle loss and resultant burden to the renal system. When glucose and fat sources are burnt, the waste products are just carbon dioxide and water, which are sent out of the body by breathing. Muscle loss generates other waste products that are to be eliminated by kidneys, which have a limited capacity for the job. Kidneys can handle the normal day-to-day waste generation but not the high toxic loads of crash dieting.

In some other studies, it was seen among obese people with heart disease that the mortality rates increase with reduction of BMI. Doctors are unable to explain this odd advantage of being obese in heart patients and call it obesity paradox. But human body is too complex a machine and human life even more complex to fully understand or explain.

My final conclusion was that I should never try to lose weight by denying food to my body. I should have my regular food with sufficient quantities of proteins, fats and carbohydrates together with vitamins and minerals. But I should try to eat less and regularly exercise.

One thing I could succeed was to start taking my tea and coffee without sugar. It did make a substantial difference because I was taking coffee or tea several times a day. A tea spoon or two in each cup would add up to hundreds of calories. Though it was difficult in the beginning, I got used to it easily soon. It felt much better as it was light on my body. Coffee with sugar now is cloying to me.

Hunger Mechanism

It is universally accepted that the most important reason for unwanted weight gain is taking in more food than we actually need. But why do we eat more than we need? Obviously, because we feel hungry! Very hungry! Ravenously hungry! Why do we feel so hungry? It is because, the body activates hunger mechanism. Why does the body activate hunger mechanism to make us to feel hungry more than the required extent? Is this all due to faulty metabolic mechanism? Or is it because of bad eating habits? Is it lack of will power? Or is it because of the food itself? Coming back to the issue, what is right quantity of food? Is it possible to calculate calorific value of food and eat correct quantity? Even if we have a mechanism to calculate calories, how is it possible to assess how much of it is absorbed and assimilated in to the body? How much of the food consumed is eaten up by the gut microbes that grow in huge numbers and pass out of the gut through the feces? (In the process the microbes do produce some very useful substances like short chain amino acids which are absorbed by the body. It is almost impossible to estimate the calorific value of such substances) Why do some people eat less and some eat more than others? Why do some voracious eaters remain thin and some people are fatty with just normal eating? There are no easy answers for these questions. There are only generalized conclusions, rough calculations and approximate values.

Though gluttony and sloth are believed by many to be the main reasons for unwanted weight gain and obesity, Dr. Robert Lustig (more about Dr. Lustig in Chapter 13) objects to such assumption. He doesn't accept treating an obese person as a perpetrator of the crime of obesity. Dr. Lustig wants to treat him instead as a victim, a victim of processed food and sugar. No one chooses to be obese, more so a five year old child. Child obesity was rare until 1980s. It is now growing because we are generously feeding children with sugar (sucrose) and high fructose corn syrup (HFCS) either directly or as added sweetener and preservative in sodas, fruit juices and several processed foods, proves Dr. Lustig with his convincing research and arguments.

Coming back to my problem, after regular observation of eating different types of foods, different quantities, at different times and in different conditions I am of the opinion that mechanism of my hunger sensation is imperfect. It makes me eat more than I need. If I am very hungry I end up eating much more than I am comfortable with. The mechanism is imperfect because the human body has not evolved enough to face the onslaught of rich, sugary, fried and fibre-free food on the metabolism. Evolution is a slow process spread over millennia, whereas changes in our food habits have taken place too fast in the past one century and especially in the past few decades. There is a serious mismatch between the type of food we eat and the process of digestion, absorption and assimilation. This mismatch might be making my hunger mechanism imperfect.

My experience of several trials suggests that eating small portions several times instead of a few big portions a day helps in several ways. It gives continuous supply of just enough energy to the body as is done in 'Just-In-Time' (JIT) concept of inventory management in manufacturing. JIT Manufacturers rely on logistics to supply them raw material required in the production cycle as and when it is required without necessitating keeping stocks of inventory in warehouses. The JIT concept is most appropriate for our eating too. It is recommended for people with diabetes too.

When we eat more high calorie food, it results in a glut of glucose in the blood. The pancreas over reacts and frantically releases more insulin, thereby bringing down the blood sugar to starvation levels. When blood sugar is low, the brain rings alarm bells for activating the hunger mechanism. That makes us hungry and drives us to eat again. Consuming large amount of high calorie food results in another problem too; it is burden on the metabolic system.

There is yet another problem with eating more. The stomach accommodates whatever we eat by extending and bulging like a balloon. Such over-eating regularly over a period makes the stomach permanently sagging and big as it loses its elasticity. You eat more; you end up eating more and more. The stomach sac keeps getting larger and larger. It becomes a limp and inelastic sac. A big sack needs to be filled with more food. We will not be satisfied unless we eat more. Sagging of stomach is also one of the factors in hunger and satiety mechanism. On the other hand if you train your body to contend with less, it just gets used to it. You will be satiated with less food.

Contradicting this concept of several small meals

a day Dr. David Sinclair (more about Dr. Sinclair in Chapter 13) suggests that we progressively limit our number of meals to increase our daily fasting time by constricting the eating window. He suggests skipping of either breakfast or dinner. He says that the human body regularly faced hunger for millennia. Hunger, like physical exercise, is a beneficial stressor to the body. A stressor prepares the body to repair and rejuvenate itself for good health and longevity.

The mechanism of hunger, appetite and satiety works at different levels. Both brain and alimentary canal work to control the sensations. A complex system of neural signals and hormones works to tell you when to eat and when to say enough. But it appears that the system is not fully understood yet.

At one level muscles and receptors in your stomach control the mechanism. The muscles of your stomach, when the sac is empty and flat, start contractions that give the hunger pangs to you. The stomach also has stretch receptors on its walls which send neural signals to the brain saying that you have had enough. But these receptors send the signal to the brain only when you have filled your stomach to the full. Contradicting this explanation, there are a few cases where people continued to have hunger pangs even after the stomach was surgically removed altogether due to cancer.

At another level two hormones leptin and ghrelin work by their fluctuating balances to control the hunger and satiety mechanisms. When you consume food your body produces leptin that reaches the brain, which in turn gives the feeling of satiety. Leptin is produced mainly by adipose tissues and enterocytes in the small intestines. When the levels of leptin in the body come down - which happens a few hours after eating - a secondary hormone, ghrelin is released, triggered by the low levels of leptin. Ghrelin makes you hungry and motivates you to eat. The production of ghrelin stops when stomach is stretched by food.

At yet another level insulin and cholecystokinin (CCK) are involved in the mechanism indirectly. Insulin is produced to regulate blood glucose levels. When glucose levels in the blood go up, insulin is produced to help the body tissues to absorb glucose. It also encourages storage of glucose as glycogen in the liver and muscles and stimulates a process called lipogenesis, which is nothing but creation of fat in fat cells. But if the level of insulin is a little more - as in the case of sudden spike of blood sugar due to taking in of food with high Glycemic Index – it brings down blood glucose to alarmingly low levels. Low levels of blood glucose ring hunger bells. It seems that while insulin by itself suppresses appetite, its effect on blood sugar triggers it. But on the other hand insulin levels in obese people are known to be high. That does not make them less hungry! The effect of insulin resistance in obese people seems to dominate the appetite suppressing trait of insulin.

Cholecystokinin (CCK) is a hormone that stimulates release of digestive enzymes and bile juice. The release of the hormone aids digestion thereby supplying glucose, amino acids and fatty acids in to the blood stream. Sufficient presence of these macronutrients gives the feeling of satiety. CCK is a known hunger suppressant.

One more chemical, serotonin is also known to play a role in appetite. Serotonin is a neurotransmitter with several functions. It is best known as mood enhancer. Its presence is known to help in attaining easy satiety. Conversely its reduced levels are linked to cravings.

It appears that a complicated and multilayered control system for hunger and satiety is evolved in humans because of the varied and omnivorous food habits. The food varied between low calorie leaves to high calorie nuts, bulky roots to densely packed eggs, sweet-sour fruits to fatty meat and from fresh milk to fermented beverages. A complicated combination of foods needed a complex system of controls.

Prasadam Effect

Yet another reason for my inability to manage my weight was the regular availability at home of *Laddu Prasadam* (a sweet offering at the Hindu religious ceremonies and prayers) of two big temples. *Kanipakam Temple*, the abode of *Lord Sri Varasiddi Vinayaka* was very close to the place of my work and we were bankers to the temple. *Tirumala-Tirupathi Temple*, the abode of

Lord Sri Venkateswara also known as *Lord Balaji* and one of the most sacred of all *Hindu Temples* was within an hour's drive. Any relative or a friend from my large circle visiting the temples would also visit us and gift us the *Laddu Prasadam* from the temples. My fondness for sweets made me eat the *Laddu* almost every day. It being sacred, even my wife who would always give a disapproving look when I ate any sweets, would not mind my eating the *Laddu*. Preventing me from eating the sacred *Laddu* would be tantamount to insulting the Lord Himself! And I was too happy to eat. Eat and gain weight!

Laddu, specifically that of the *Tirumala -Tirupathi* Temple, treated as most sacred is also one of the tastiest of all sweets. Made of *ghee* (clarified butter), *jaggery* (condensed sugarcane juice), Chick Pea flour, dry fruits, nuts and many other aromatic spices, the sacred and delicious *Laddu* is a popular and customary gift. A joke in the business circles was that even the toughest and most incorruptible of the Government Officers could be 'tamed' with a gift of *Tirupathi Laddu*. It was sacrilegious to refuse and too delicious and tempting not to accept. Once the gift was accepted the receiver was obliged to be kind hearted to the giver!

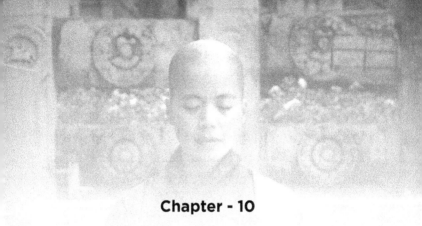

Chapter - 10

Another Relocation

One more transfer took me to a far off town in the North West region of the country. I had to live alone away from my wife and children at the new place as I was transferred in the middle of an academic year. My children could not be admitted in the school at the new place in the mid year. I was angry at my transfer and was almost frustrated. But what could not be cured had to be endured. I, however, had to accept later about what Shakespeare says in "As You Like It": 'Sweet are the uses of adversity'.

Once I joined at the new place, I was initially very unhappy and disappointed for one more reason also. I found that the state of affairs at the office were not at all good. The computer systems supplied by the Head Office for computerizing bank operations were not even unpacked. The work was heavy and I did not see any hope of maintaining my exercise program. All the branch heads who worked till then never lived in the town. It was said that they used to 'live out of a suit case'; they would stay in hotels from Monday to Friday and go home regularly, to their family in the metropolitan city. Service to customers was not of my standards. Employees had a very low morale. It was necessary to change things to suit my work as well as me.

I stopped all my walking and exercises for about two months and started 24x7 data entry work by involving everybody, security guards included, in whatever capacity possible and accepting whatever little they could contribute, for computerizing the bank transactions. My hard work paid good dividends and all the new systems were in place. I became relatively free in the evenings due to computerization. The time-consuming daily, weekly and monthly balancing work was taken care of by the computers. Even the Management Information System Reports were easy to prepare, thanks to the easy availability of data.

I found out that there was a good club in the town with a gym and swimming pool at a nominal fee for officers and managers who came on transfers. I started my workouts on a regular basis. My swimming sessions were enjoyable.

Swimming without any reservations is the best form of all exercises. It exercises many muscle groups. Unlike in walking or running, the weight of the body is not borne by the hips, knees and ankles. The buoyancy of water is very gentle on the body. It is the most suitable exercise to start with for obese or overweight people. Regular swimming gives you a supple and lithe body.

But unfortunately for me it wasn't possible to sustain my exercise in water for long. I was inclined to relax the moment I entered water. I would float and enjoy in the cool environment of the pool after a few laps. I was reluctant to leave the pool soon enough. I stopped swimming too as it was affecting my other exercises. I would enter the pool occasionally to relax in the cool water.

My workout program in the gym was very successful. Six days a week, I would walk for 20 minutes on the treadmill, bicycle or do skipping for 20 minutes and later did strength training also for about 20 minutes. I continued *Yogasanams* 2-3 times a week at home. Within a few months and for the first time in my life and after nearly a decade of serious efforts I was fit. I was feeling fit and looking fit. I was congratulated by many of my friends. My stamina and strength were good. I had a BMI of 25. I was agile.

An over-heard comment of an insurance advisor, one day, pleased and assured me beyond doubt that I was quite fit. I had purchased a life insurance policy. The insurance company was insisting that I get a medical certificate from a hospital in a nearby city as a precondition for issuing the insurance policy. But I wanted the insurer to exempt me from that hassle. While trying to convince his senior officer that he argued in Hindi interspersed with English. "No need, Sir. He may be in his mid-forties, but he is fit as a fiddle. You should see him move around in his office. You will easily be convinced".

My people back home were quite pleased that I was healthy and fit though alone in a far off place. Many of my old friends wondered how I could 'achieve' my fitness and started asking advice too!

Happiness Program

While maintaining my hard earned fitness I continued to try any new opportunity that I came across for the upkeep of my fitness and health. The Art of Living Foundation (ALF), a non-profit international humanitarian organization based in Bengaluru, South India, conducted a basic course called 'Happiness Program' near my work place. ALF, founded by spiritual teacher and an ambassador of peace, Sri Sri Ravi Shankar, works with an objective of stress-free and violence free world by rekindling of human values.

The program teaches *dhyanam, pranayamam* and some basic *yogasanams*. '*Sudarshan Kriya*', a simple breathing technique is their specialty. The courses have programs to inculcate Positive Mental Attitude (PMA) in the participants and help people to develop good interpersonal relations. Though it was an excellent course for beginners, I did not personally find anything new to learn. I was already practicing most of what they were teaching. One another minor negative feature of the ALF that I did not like was the excessive personality cult that the teachers and some followers tried to create around the founder.

One interesting observation I made a note of at the Art of Living basic course was that some participants experienced a sort of 'runner's high'(More about Runner's High in Chapter 17) after '*Sudarshan Kriya*'; a series of fast, normal and slow breathing activity. It was something puzzling to me for I knew that only some experienced runners - not all but a few - get the 'high' after a very physically exhausting aerobic event like a marathon. But here was a case where an activity - that was hardly demanding, leave alone exhausting - caused the 'high'. I confirmed from the course instructor that they did get such cases occasionally.

The only thing common between a marathon runner and a '*Sudarshan Kriya*' practitioner is the intense activity of lungs, abdominal muscles and the diaphragm, a sheet of muscle which separates thoracic and abdominal cavities in the body. 'Runner's High' seems to be a rare occurrence in both. It is for the physiologists and neurologists to see any link here.

Other Fitness Lessons

Meanwhile I was also observing and learning whatever I could about health and fitness. I was discussing with anybody who was interested in the subject. The experience of two of my friends enlightened me about the complexity, uniqueness and unpredictable nature of human body. A fellow fitness enthusiast in my gym, whom I call my FFE, was very regular to his exercises. He was a tall but overweight young man, otherwise handsome. He was an eligible bachelor. He used to work out regularly with free weights and would also do the aerobic exercises on the treadmill. His sole aim was to bring down his weight. Being slim, he reasoned, was a ticket to get a beautiful wife. But he was struggling with his weight as all his efforts were not giving results. He was getting disappointed. Meanwhile his employer, an American Multinational Company, running a power generation plant, came out with an attractive incentive scheme to encourage employees to walk. The health promoting incentive was a cute little waist-belt worn pedometer. The device was distributed to all employees with a condition. It would be treated as a gift from the company if the employee recorded a daily average of 5000 steps for a period of three months. All those who did not reach the target had to return the pedometer to the company. My FFE being very enthusiastic set himself a target of 10000 steps and would walk at every opportunity in the sprawling power plant. And in the process, his bulk melted away, literally! He did get a beautiful young lady as his wife in the next one year.

My FFE's experience was a lesson to me. The walking 'workout', if it could be called one, is hardly a strenuous exercise. Even in terms of calorie spend it would not be much when compared with his treadmill and gym workouts. But what seemed to be the difference was the activity being spread over the whole day. The muscles of the body were in fat-burning mode most of the day. It also struck to my mind that many thin people known to me were almost invariably very physically active individuals. Such people would not sit at one place even for a few minutes. They move around in homes and offices for every small work and errand with least dependence on others. It seems to be fairly clear to me now that frequent physical activity during the day is good for weight loss. It should be equivalent to moderate exercise of 2 or 3 even more sessions of 20-30 minute each. Such activity keeps the body in enhanced fat burning mode for hours after the exercise and helps to reduce fat and body weight.

Another experience was that of a customer of my bank whom I name as The Art of Living Foundation (ALF) Beneficiary. He was a portly middle aged man with a friendly smile. He was an occasional visitor to the bank as most of his bank work was looked after by his assistants. It was a surprise to find him very thin suddenly one day. He didn't appear to be sick. He was his usual cheerful self except that he was looking different due to the loss of fat under the facial skin.

I was initially hesitant to ask the ALF Beneficiary about his sudden changed appearance as it was too personal a matter to enquire. But I had to yield to my curiosity as it was too interesting a matter to ignore. I called him over phone and asked him to share a cup of tea as well as the secret of his success with me. He readily obliged. While the effect of what he did was astounding to me, the cause was more. He explained that he was continuing with his daily two mile walk as before. The cause of his weight loss seemed to be his breathing exercises he was practicing which he had learnt in The Art of Living Foundation's basic course. He had had a health check up too to rule out any health problems. It was very amazing to learn that a simple alternating fast and slow breathing exercise could burn fat off the body of a man. Though thousands of people practice breathing exercises and *Sudarshan Kriya* regularly, it is rare to find people who lose much of their weight. But strange and unique as it is, it happened in the case of TAL Beneficiary. A simple breathing exercise could fire up intense metabolic activity to burn fat.

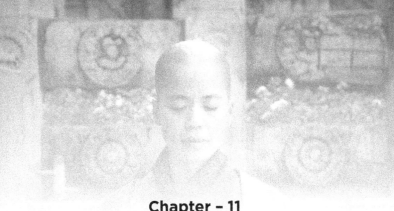

Chapter – 11

My Personality

Whether it was my simple village background or my family's good bringing up or my reading of good books or my association with some kind people or might be all of these, I had somehow developed a Positive Mental Attitude (PMA) with most of its ingredients - optimism, hope, tolerance, empathy, kindliness, generosity, integrity, faith, courage and initiative. I never had to worry about interpersonal relations and could get along with all sorts of people. But all that had its negative side too. Some PMA traits would work against me and my goals.

I have to admit here that I lacked a few positive qualities that are required in life for success. They are; tact, ability to project myself and firmness of a decision.

In this world of competition one has to maneuver through the crowd of the society carefully but tactfully making the way and ultimately reaching the goal. The moving forward should be such that every available opportunity is taken advantage of without jostling the way and with no hint of being selfish. But my empathetic attitude would make me to make way for others instead of making the way for myself. I need to expend more time and resources to get what could otherwise easily be got with tact.

The competition in general is so high and the competitors are so many that an organization or the society cannot sift and choose. So only a person who climbs up a pedestal and cries out, projects himself and seeks attention would be noticed. An unassuming and humble person remains unrecognized. Modesty is at a disadvantage now or may not be a virtue any more.

Inability to stand firm in the face of pleading by others with their problems is another issue. Striking a balance between kindliness and firmness in a decision is difficult. Again I end up spending more time, money and other resources to satisfy my kindliness, empathy and generosity. It is expensive and hard work to maintain one's PMA. But trying to change and adopt an attitude not natural to my personality would be disastrous and my life would be miserable. I therefore continue to be as positive and as good a human being as ever, how hard or how expensive it might be. It is good for my health!

Positive attitude seems to be an essential quality of fitness. A study reported a few years ago in a magazine quotes that negative attitude leads to depression. Depression in turn is linked to increased death rate due to heart disease. A Gerontologist from USA led a team who followed nearly three thousand people who were old or in late middle age for four years. It was found at the end of the study that people with major depression had 300% more risk of death due to heart disease than those who were not depressed. People with mild depression also had a 50% higher risk than normal people.

It is believed that negative attitude and depression lead to stress and stress triggers release of increased amounts of hormone cortisol, which causes higher heart rate and high blood pressure. Depression and resultant stress also lead to other negative effects such as lethargy, reduced mobility and lack of control over food consumption.

The good side of PMA made me a good friend to many and a desirable colleague wherever I worked. My fitness and good health enabled me to work hard and work efficiently. My work showed good results in business growth and good performance in other parameters of my bank work. It earned me the 'Best Manager' award too.

Idea of Writing a Book

I got the idea of writing down my experience and experiments in the form of a book because I was successfully managing my weight and fitness. I had started noting down briefly what I ate and what I did each day for managing my hyper acidity. I continued recording my exercise schedules also. But I was not sure if writing at that stage was appropriate. My intention was to write the experiences and achievements of a layman, not about a professional athlete or a sports person. A professional has time and resources at his disposal to maintain his fitness. A coach in a gym or an athlete training for a track and field competition is fit by default. Their job is to work out and train. An athlete or a sportsman is motivated to control his food intake. He has incentives for being in 'form'. It is no great a deal for him to be fit.

The circumstances under which I attained my fitness were also similar to that of an athlete. I did not have much house hold responsibility as I was living alone while my wife back home was caring for my children in high school finals. Free from drudgery of manual accounting, I was quite comfortable managing my office. So time was at my disposal!

My residence, my office and my club with gym and swimming pool were all within a one-kilometre range. I could entrust a work like monthly report preparation to my junior officers in late the evenings, go to the gym for a work out and get back to office for signing the reports before the courier pick-up time.

One more aspect of my life at that time in favour of fitness was my food intake. The Gujarati food in restaurants and hotels, at least initially, was not at all palatable to my South Indian taste buds. I had no choice but to learn and start cooking my own food. Though I took great care in making my food varied enough to be nutritious with vegetables, eggs, meat and milk products, it was not the sumptuous and tasty meal that I was used to at home. I was just eating so that I lived and lived healthy. I had not controlled my food intake by will power. I was forced to reduce my consumption by the circumstances of my living. It was clear to me that I was greatly 'favored' by my living and working conditions in reaching my fitness goals. Could that be sustained in any changed circumstances? I was doubtful. So I wanted to wait for some more time to write my book. The wait extended to more than a decade.

Yet Another Transfer - Early Retirement

The next transfer and a promotion brought me to a metropolitan city nearer home. There was a beautiful park for walking and a gym available near my home. But I could hardly use the facilities. I had to spend more than two hours of the day for commuting to work. The work at the bank was heavy and I was short of time most of the days. My daily morning exercise routine was the first casualty of my heavy work and long commute. More over I had to pass through the crowded and dusty commercial area of the city to reach office. Whether it was because of the stress of the office work and commuting or pollution of the city, I was hungry very often. I had to have a snack in between breakfast and lunch as well as lunch and dinner.

Long hours at the office desk, stress, tiresome commute and lack of exercise were taking me back to the miserable days of my thirties. I started getting overweight again. My stamina was not as it used to be. I was getting tired and exhausted by evening and could not get up early enough even for a morning walk. I was just two years short of my fiftieth birthday.

My carefully acquired ability to work in spite of stress, my aptitude for dealing with people and some of my other traits were most suitable for the job I was doing. My bank management would keep me continuously as a branch head for years without any relief. While many fellow managers managed to get themselves posted to cosy corners of administrative offices every few years, a few people like me were continuously kept in stressful jobs without respite. There is always that much only that one can do, can bear with and manage comfortably after a certain level.

My work would not even allow me to eat on time nor was there time for exercise and relaxation. I felt that the stress was not worth bearable and had a doubt that it might lead to other serious ailments. Stress in early age may cause hyperacidity alone. But it leads to many far more dangerous ailments such as diabetes, hypertension and heart problems in later years.

It was a time to choose. A career that might be financially rewarding after a quarter century of work experience and gained seniority or good health with less money. I chose the latter and took early retirement. Just as a celebrated poet said, I took the road less travelled. That did make a difference. It was a difference for fitness, for good health and for happiness.

One interesting aspect of my feeling hungry which I noted later was that air pollution appeared to play a definite role. Whether I was physically active or not I was hungry often while in the cities. It would be worse if I went out and moved around. But if I were in my village and my farm, I would not feel hungry so often. I thought that air pollution with dust which is high in cities when compared to villages might be the reason for my problem.

I had to rethink when I realized that the problem was not there even when I was exposed to dust on hot dry days during the farming operations. Therefore it can be assumed that soil and plant based dust do not make me hungry. It appears that the automobile fumes and other urban dust seem to cause stress that in turn causes a sort of hunger. I understand that the body treats any foreign organism or a foreign dust particle as an enemy and starts preparing for a war on the enemy. If it is a known enemy - like soil dust or plant based particles I was exposed to as a child - the body already knows how to deal and hence there is no stress. If it is an unknown enemy - such as auto fumes, concrete dust and plastic dust - the body has to prepare for a full scale war. The stress caused by such preparation makes me hungry.

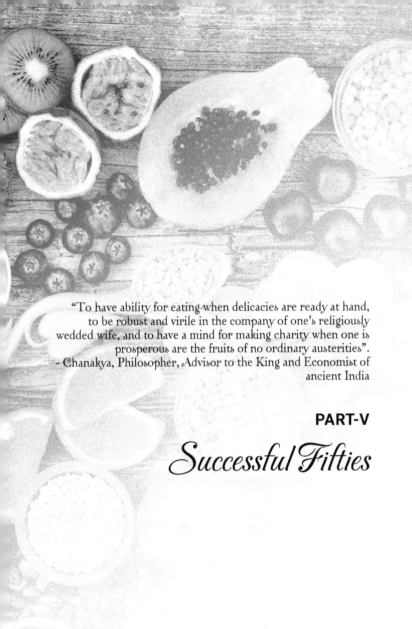

"To have ability for eating when delicacies are ready at hand, to be robust and virile in the company of one's religiously wedded wife, and to have a mind for making charity when one is prosperous are the fruits of no ordinary austerities".
- Chanakya, Philosopher, Advisor to the King and Economist of ancient India

PART-V

Successful Fifties

Chapter - 12

Vipassana

Once out of bank service I had free time. I dabbled in business for some time and finally quit that too. I started focusing more on my family's ancestral farm. It was good to be a free man. My time was in my control. I started regular exercises. I also practiced some *Yogasanams, Pranayama and Dhyanam.* It was time to do more with my fitness, health and well being.

I had learnt about Vipassana Meditation through a friend and wished to attend the course. But I could not do while I was in the bank service, because it was not possible to take a long break from work. My farming activity was flexible enough to allow me to attend such a course. The beginner residential course needs a complete 10 day cut-off from the outside world. As a participant you will not have access to television, newspapers, books or phones. No personal contact with others is possible. The participants are strictly instructed on the first day itself not to talk to each other. You have to maintain a 'noble silence'; not just maintaining total silence, you should also not communicate with others by any means. No sign language, no eye contact, not even wishing each other by smiling. The only person you can talk to, only in whispers, is the teacher and that is for clarifying any doubts regarding the meditation technique.

Vipassana is a system of meditation popularized mainly by the visionary master, S N Goenka, who is now known to many as "The Man who taught the World to Meditate". Vipassana is a very simple system originally said to have been discovered and perfected by Gautama Buddha. It is non-sectarian and people of any faith or even non-believers can follow. The system uses the whole body to achieve a meditative state that can be sustained long enough. All other forms of meditation involve an image or an object or a color or a sound to focus and meditate. In these types of meditation it is extremely difficult to focus for long without diversion. But in Vipassana system, you are trained and made to feel the sensations or pulsations arising naturally within the body. You start the training by first being aware of the breath through the nostrils. It is called Ana-pana. You are then made to feel the flow of air by the inner walls of nostrils.

The continuous focus on the flow of air through the nostrils will slowly make you realize that there are vibrations or pulsations in the inner walls of your nose.

Once that is achieved you have entered the world of Vipassana! The teacher, masterfully and step by step, makes you to be aware of the pulsations in every part, every square inch of the body – outside and inside. The pulsations last as long as you observe and pass as soon as you shift your focus on another area or part. You have to merely observe the sensations with your mind and learn not to react to them.

It is said that the Vipassana, also called 'mindfulness meditation' guides you to attain a balanced mind, clears the mind of any impurities and helps you to get rid of the extremes of feelings and thus make you lead a happy life. The master assures that your conversion will be from misery to happiness, from ignorance to wisdom and from bondage to liberation. It is known to help one to overcome feelings of greed, avarice, anger, infatuation and eliminate anxiety, agitation, nervousness and stress. Vipassana is also known to cure migraines.

While it is difficult for me to judge and quantify the benefits mentioned above, I found other benefits of *Vipassana* Meditation that are perceptible to me. Within a few minutes of being in meditation, my breathing is automatically deep and continuous. My mind is free from wavering thoughts. I get totally refreshed after my meditation. I can clearly feel the state of serenity and peace and quiet. And I am happier than before.

One amusing experience in attending the Vipassana course and practicing the meditation is how you are trained to ignore itches. When you are slowly getting in to the process of meditation, you are frequently disturbed by itching. When you have the urge to scratch you are advised and trained not to react. Surprisingly, the itch disappears. If you ignore regularly for some time they completely disappear. Symbolically speaking, life's small 'itches' will go away if you ignore them. The lesson is not to react to every small irritant of life.

It was always intriguing to me about what makes meditation so effective. How is that none can dispute the benefits of meditation? How does it work? It is universally experienced that meditation is the best stress buster. Meditation is also known to improve (lower) heart rate, lower blood pressure and improve breathing. It helps to boost immunity too. For many people meditation provides relief from pain. But how does it work? Neurologists and scientists are yet to fully explain.

The common characteristics of most mediators I have come across are:

- They are cool and balanced
- They have clarity of thought
- They are happy and often very contended
- They are healthier than most people of their age
- They live, in my opinion, longer too

The obvious reasons that I see for the effectiveness of the meditation practice are:

1. Continuous and trained focus on the object of meditation diverts one completely from any agitation that is there on the mind and gives relief from stress.

2. An unwavering focus and un-agitated mind help the body to breathe deep. Deep breathing in turn leads to better circulation of oxygenated blood, good health and high energy levels. This can be observed in people who don't meditate but have the ability to be totally involved and concentrated in whatever they do. No amount of work tires them. They are just as fresh at the end of a demanding work day as they are in the morning. One who has such ability can aptly be called a *karma-yogi*.

3. The very process of meditation is voluntary control of mind to concentrate on anything that can give clarity of thought.

4. Meditation is also known to help in production of endorphins and serotonin. Endorphins are known to give relief from pain and serotonin helps in stabilization of mood, feeling of well-being and happiness.

Dr. Bernard Lown (1921-2021), Lithuanian-American Cardiologist, inventor of heart defibrillator and one of the founders of an antiwar group, Physicians for Peace that won the Nobel Peace Prize has a convincing explanation for the Chinese traditional acupuncture's efficacy. He mentions an incident in his book *The Lost Art of Healing* about how he got instant relief from his severe back pain with acupuncture during a visit to China. He explains in the book that the tiny nerve endings under the skin get stimulated by acupuncture to produce neuro-chemicals that act as pain relievers. My inference is that the same stimulation works in *Vipassana* meditation too. I systematically feel the stimulation like 'pulse' all over the body while meditating. The difference between acupuncture and *Vipassana* is that in case of acupuncture the nerve endings are stimulated by external pins and in *Vipassana* it is self stimulation generated internally.

My Sleep

Other than the days I suffered disturbed sleep when I overdid my exercising, I used to sleep well. I learnt over a period to avoid overdoing any exercise and always slept well, or so I thought. It is only after I started wearing a smart watch much later that I truly learnt to differentiate a good sleep from a bad one. The Fitbit smart watch that I use (its functions explained in Chapter 15) showed the flaws in my sleeping habits. Here is what I learnt about sleep:

- The best medicine for good sleep is a physically tired body. Exercise is only one part. If you work hard, any type of work without taking the metal stress, you will sleep very well.

- Excessive exercise, as already explained disturbs sleep. Exercising close to bed time also disturbs sleep.

- Relaxing before bed time gives you quality sleep. It helps to have memory and brain function boosting Rapid Eye Movement (REM) sleep.

- Eating late in the night is a big enemy of sleep. Your late dinner will make your cardiovascular and pulmonary system to continue to work even during their rest time. You may sleep, but it would be poor quality sleep. If sleep has to be of good quality, your sleeping heart rate (SHR) has to be mostly less than your resting heart rate (RHR). Food in the stomach demands a higher heart rate.

- Having a heavy dinner or eating food rich in calories, drinking caffeinated beverages and taking alcohol also have the same effect as having late dinner. Shakespeare's quote from Macbeth, "it provokes the desire, but it takes away the performance" is very relevant for alcohol on sleep. Alcohol makes one sleepy but the sleep quality is poor.

One interesting contradiction that we see is about the rejuvenating stressors on body as proposed by Dr. David Sinclair (explained in Chapter 13). Dr. Sinclair is of the opinion that stressing the body with hunger, exercise, heat and cold help the body to repair and rejuvenate itself and keep it healthy. But how about sleep deprivation? Is it not a good stressor? "No", says Dr. Sinclair, "It is an exception!" The damage to the body caused by sleep deprivation is worse! Good sleep favours the body with spurts of growth hormone production. Growth hormone is an essential chemical produced by the body during sleep and it is helpful for the body for several functions, including for proper maintenance and repair of the body tissues.

Unusual Pain in My Foot

'Plantar Fasciitis' was the diagnosis made by the Orthopedic Surgeon. A strange name with two consecutive 'i's, I was initially wondering if it was mis-spelt by the doctor. But I was wrong. It was 'Plantar Fasciitis', correctly spelt.

I had severe pain in my left foot. It started a few months after I started looking after my mango garden. I had got the garden fenced with barbed wire and began clearing, pruning and ploughing operations in the orchard. I was actively involved in supervising and also once in a while participating in the work. I could move about the orchard with the same energy of a regular farmer. I was quite happy and proud of myself that I could withstand the physical strain of the work of a whole day even in oppressively hot weather.

The pain I got was unusual because a pain generally subsides with rest and aggravates without. But in my case, I would get it if I rested my feet. I would have difficulty standing soon after I got up from bed. It would subside after a while if I moved around. There would not be any pain as long as I was physically active and on my feet. The pain would reappear soon after a little rest. The relief from preliminary treatment with pain relievers, support braces and rest was temporary. I had to seek a professional's help.

My visit to Orthopedic Surgeon and the diagnosis made me very curious about the problem and the reasons for my getting it. I learnt that the pain was because of the inflammation of fascia, the tough band of tissue that connects my heel bone to the base of the toes. What was surprising for me was that I did not have any of the risk factors, as noted in the medical literature, for the problem. I was not excessively over weight, had neither flat feet nor high arch. I did not change foot wear; leave alone an abrupt change of foot wear with high heels to flat heels. I did not agree with and ruled out one possible factor given by doctors - being on feet for long hours - because I was doing that for months; personally supervising erection of a few kilometers of barbed wire fence, clearing the mango garden of tall weeds, pruning over five thousand mango plants and finally ploughing.

It was when I was wondering about the cause of my unusual pain at home one day that my sister-in-law guessed the most appropriate cause of my plantar fasciitis. She told me out of her own experience that my problem might be because of my walking in the ploughed fields. The last major activity in the orchard before the starting of my pain was ploughing, which made the ground uneven throughout. My walking on the uneven ground disturbed my plantar fascia! My walking in the ploughed field was more like changing my foot-wear from high heels to flat soles - and even the very opposite of high heels - with every step of my walking.

My feet had got used to move around on mirror polished marble slabs and smooth tiles, walking on bitumen or concrete roads or rubber lined tread mill. Sudden change to moving around in the field was bearable. But, to walk in ploughed field - my feet could not take any more!

Plantar Fasciitis is generally, the doctors say, a 'self-limiting' condition, which means it resolves on its own. The condition may not have any long term harmful effect on your health. My pain disappeared, just as the doctor said, very soon.

Once you attain a comfortable fitness level, it is advisable to walk some days on uneven ground too. The small and not so small stones pressing against your sole stimulate the body. A small pothole like dip in the ground or a small heap of soil in a field can pressurize different spots and all corners in the joints of the hip, knee, ankle, foot and toes. This helps to give differential stress on the body and trains it to be agile and to keep good balance.

Balancing is the ability of your body to right itself when you stumble. It helps you to keep upright, walk or do other daily activities. You take balancing for granted because it is instinctively done by your body. It is in fact done by a complex interaction of different organs of the body. Your eyes, vestibular system in your ears, nerve receptors called proprioceptors in feet and joints communicate with the brain and make subtle movements in the legs to keep you upright.

Your ability to balance is an integral part of your fitness and is an asset in old age. If you are fit, your muscles will respond promptly to the commands of the brain and keep you upright. Your strength and balance will help you to stand firm in spite of a trip-over on an unnoticed cable on the floor or a misstep on an uneven ground. A good balance aids you in preventing falls that can lead to injuries and fractures.

The present day comforts, conveniences and smooth life have impaired our ability to balance ourselves though we inherit a body that is designed to have an excellent ability to balance itself. We walk and move on even and smooth surfaces. There is never an opportunity for the body to test its balancing ability and keep itself in form. It becomes almost dysfunctional as we age. An aged body cannot withstand a sudden jerk or a tripping or a slip or a necessity to dodge something like a youthful body. The result is a fall leading to fractures.

My Cholesterol and Sugar

While I managed to be fit, I continued to be slightly overweight all along. I could not fully get rid of the weight gained by me just before my taking early retirement. My regular blood tests showed that both my cholesterol and sugar levels were within normal range. But they were always on the border of the higher limits. My aim was to maintain both cholesterol and sugar by regular exercise and controlled food. Though I was not as bad as in my thirties and forties, I was a bad dieter nonetheless. I would not miss or could not resist an opportunity to eat sweets or unhealthy snacks when I attended parties and feasts or even at home if my wife forgot to hide them from me.

One of the routine blood tests showed a sudden drop of cholesterol to a healthy level. The repeat test also showed reduced levels. I was puzzled at the reduced cholesterol as my body weight remained as before. There was no change in my workout schedule too. I realized that I had been physically very active during the previous two months. I had installed new drip lines for irrigation in my mango garden. I was regularly checking the drippers, kneeling down or squatting, at each plant to ensure that they are dripping. I was also exposed to the sunlight for quite long each day. I learnt a lesson that the whole day physical activity is the key and so is exposure to sunlight. Both physical activity and sun light are a part of human life. Denying these to the body is inviting disease. In an experiment in Australia, 10 middle aged overweight Australian Aborigines suffering from type 2 diabetes were asked to return to hunter gatherer lifestyle. After period of just seven weeks their diabetes got completely reversed.

I also did an experiment with my cholesterol level while I was just managing to be on the border for both cholesterol and sugar. I had read an article on health that said that, it is the carbohydrate that is responsible for increase in cholesterol. The article also hinted that denying enough fats to the body may also induce the body to produce more cholesterol. I was very curious to know and personally experiment. I started to have two eggs together with the yolk - either boiled or as omelet - a day for breakfast along with a small cup of boiled lentils. My lunch and dinner remained unchanged. The duration and intensity of my exercises also remained the same. My weight check and blood tests after two months did not surprise me. My weight went up slightly. But my cholesterol level came down to normal. What I read was right!

The weight gain could be explained with the increase in calorie intake. The coming down of cholesterol could be explained only with fat intake. Healthy fats are not bad at all. Thereafter I started taking an egg a day regularly.

My fasting sugar levels which were within normal range during the first half of my fifties started slightly northward in my mid fifties. I was expecting it all along for two valid reasons. First, I had a family history of diabetes. Second, my food habits were bad enough.

The fasting glucose reading was in the 120-125 mg/dl range. My contention was that it was pre-diabetes and that I could try and control with diet and exercise. All the doctors in my family and extended family - qualified and experienced, qualified but not experienced and those studying to be qualified - were not convinced with my argument. Their contention was that the pre-diabetes range for Asians was under 110 and so I had no choice but to use medicines. Their further convincing point was that the wonder drug, 'metformin' was harmless and was prescribed as a safe drug even for obesity. I had to finally yield and started using a metformin dose of 250mg/day. The fasting sugar levels, as well as postprandial, came down to normal very soon. There was no problem with the use of medicine. There were no side effects. It was just fine.

But I was not happy using medicines on a regular basis. I had read that diabetes was reversible and I wanted to reverse mine. I changed my food from rice to coarse grains. I stopped taking all flour based food and sweets on six of the seven days in a week. I took specific care to take balanced diet with vegetables, cheese, eggs and nuts. And, I intensified my exercises. My weight came down and I was really fit again. I stopped my metformin tablet for a week and went for a blood test. My fasting and postprandial blood sugar was normal. My diabetes was reversed! I repeated the tests after three more 'no medicine' months. Yes, confirmed, my diabetes was reversed!

My carefully managed sugar and cholesterol reappeared as a problem during Covid-19 pandemic lockdowns. A combination of factors forced on me by the pandemic, I believe, led to this problem. Reduced mobility, deviation from millet food, lack of exposure to sun light and plantar fasciitis in my right foot, necessitating rest from exercise, led to my higher than normal blood sugar and cholesterol. I was forced to use medicines that helped to bring down both sugar and cholesterol dramatically to normal levels. I experimented by stopping the cholesterol drug and also totally avoiding sugar in my food for a month to test Dr. Robert Lustig's (more about Dr. Lustig in Chapter 13) recommendation. It worked well for me, though the results were not as dramatic as in using medicine. But, contradicting my experiment, the cholesterol levels of my 78-year old brother-in-law were absolutely normal in spite of his regular use of sugar in several cups of sugary coffee that he consumes every day. He takes medicines though to control his blood glucose. It may be that he, being a slim farmer who did hard physical work throughout his life, has high capacity to process the harmful fructose in the sugar that he consumes. It could also be due to the efficacy of his diabetes drugs in controlling his cholesterol too.

I continue to use metformin, which is prescribed by my doctors for controlling my blood glucose. Metformin works, as Dr. David Sinclair (topic on Dr. Sinclair in Chapter 13) says, as a longevity drug and helps to postpone or altogether prevent many age related ailments.

Nature of Food We Eat Today

The starchy and highly refined food that most of us consume now is processed to such a fine extent that the body can almost absorb the small particles directly into the blood stream with minimum digestion process. The food that most of the people eat today is almost free from fibre. The human body was designed by evolution. The digestive system and metabolic system are compatible with hand pounded and cooked food but not machine processed food. Protein rich and fatty food such as milk, meat, eggs are acceptable to the body but not refined sugar. Boiling and roasting to an extent may be good but not deep fried food. The body was used to only an occasional seasonal fruit, but not fiber free sweetened fruit juice.

The evolutionary scientists hypothesize that the humans developed sweet tooth because the body needs vitamins and minerals richly available in fruits. Human beings were attracted to eating sweet and colorful fruits to get the essential vitamins, minerals and antioxidants, which remove harmful molecules from the body. But the problem with the present day fruits is that they are too sweet. The sustained efforts of smart farmers, horticultural scientists and plant breeders have selectively eliminated all but the fruits that are the sweetest. Eating more than the necessary quantity of fruit may lead to either weight gain or hyperacidity or both.

Another major challenge the modern day eating has posed to the human body is incompatibility in assimilation of food. The system is very efficient in absorbing the digested carbohydrates, proteins and fats because it was designed for getting the best out of very fibrous low calorie food. The body which was designed for coarse, hand pounded and minimally cooked low calorie food is getting machine pulverized, overcooked, almost fiber free processed food which is too rich in calories. The entire quantity of food consumed is easily available for the body soon after eating. The food absorbed has to be spent or saved for future use. Body does not need so much of carbohydrates, fats and proteins for its maintenance. Even growing children and adolescents cannot utilize so much of food because the efficient assimilation process takes in most of what is consumed and imposes enormous burden on the metabolic system.

One more problem with processed foods is that of too much of some nutrients and too little of some other. Dr. Robert Lustig (topic on Dr.Lustig in Chapter 13) repeats in most of his talks that modern diets have too much of trans-fats, omega-6 fatty acids, branched chain amino acids, alcohol and sugar all of which overload the liver. On the other hand fibre, micronutrients and omega-3 fatty acids which are anti-inflammatory are too little. Fibre which is crucial for the growth and maintenance of gut micro biome is removed for increasing the shelf life of processed foods.

Fibre in the food has several very beneficial functions;

- Fibre slows down the digestion and absorption of excess sugar there by controlling the blood sugar levels.

- It also acts as a barrier and limits the assimilation of excess nutrients and helps in body weight regulation.

- Fibre is the base on which gut microbes grow. Gut microbes produce and supply several physiologically useful substances to the body. Colon bacteria are known to digest soluble fibre and produce short chain fatty acids which are anti-inflammatory and also are insulin-suppressants.

- Fibre forms the bulk and helps easy movement out of waste from the body.

I learnt about an interesting point during a visit to a vermi-compost unit and casual talk with the farmer about the production, demand and supply of vermi-compost. He was telling that he never uses dung from commercial dairy farms because the earth worms, which chew up dung and excrete the compost, do not flourish in beds filled with dung from commercial dairy farms. It wasn't a surprise for me. Cows and buffalos are ruminants and have four-compartment stomach to digest tough grass which is full of fibre. The pulverized grain that is fed to the dairy animals in commercial dairy farms is literally a piece of cake for those ruminants. It is calorie and nutrient rich but ultra-processed food for the ruminants. The entire food is easily digested and completely assimilated. There is neither fibre to live on nor nutrients to feed on for the gut microbes. The antibiotics added to the feed kill whatever microbes that are there in the system. What comes out as 'dung' is a total waste that is unfit even for worms!

Coming back to our food, while an ordinary and regular meal of a normal house hold, full of processed, fibre free, fried and sugar filled, is so bad for the body, the food served in the feasts and parties is beyond tolerance.

There are in fact many people whose bodies face such feasts and parties day after day, every day!

Lifestyle of Most People Today

"I smoke like a chimney, drink like a fish and eat like a pig. I don't exercise…" admitted a distinguished armchair-entrepreneur and philanthropist of Mumbai, India. His reply was to a question in a newspaper interview about what made him lose sleep at night. There was a tone of utter despair in his response. This is the typical life style of many people everywhere. Life of many busy and successful people of today is one long and unending party of dinner get-togethers, wedding feasts, birth-day parties, success celebrations, new-year treats, festivals and more. It is as if these social events are deliberately designed to destroy the health of everybody who participates. The range of drinks served, the varieties of traditional food, modern foods, sweets, meat dishes, fried vegetables of different cuisines, desserts and ice-creams coupled with the bonhomie would make even a man of steel to succumb. You would end up consuming a couple of days' worth of recommended calorie intake even if you sample half of the dishes on display. Unless you go to such parties with a strong will, it is impossible not to overeat. It is high time people made a conscious decision not to overindulge in such partying.

A study reported shows that a varied menu with many dishes makes one eat more. The researchers found that those offered a varied menu consume more calories than people who were offered a simple meal. The study says it is as much as 60% more. The researchers opine that when we have a simple meal with fewer choices we tend to stop eating as soon as our hunger is satisfied. It can as well be that the fewer calories of food be the right kind like vegetables, whole grains, lentils, nuts, dairy, eggs and fruits!

When my attending wedding feasts or parties gets too frequent, I conquer my temptation to overeat by having a light meal of millets and vegetables just before I attend. It helps me to control my craving for sweets and tempting dishes!

My Present Food Habits

I now eat 3-4 varieties of raw and seasoned vegetables, a chunk of homemade cheese and any one of soaked lentils - green gram, chick pea, horse gram and cow pea – regularly for breakfast. If I forget to soak the lentils the previous evening, I boil them but take care not to over boil so that my pancreas is not stressed. I want my stomach to work hard. And of course, a boiled egg a day also is a part of my lunch or dinner. I also eat a serving of fruit every day as a snack, an hour or more before my dinner. My lunch and dinner consist of sorghum or pearl-millet *roti* (Indian bread) or rice or fox-tail millet with vegetables, *dal* (lentils) and curd regularly. Occasionally I have meat too. When I say rice or millet here they are unpolished whole grains. The rice generally sold in the market is thoroughly polished to look milky-white and pleasing to the eye. But in the process the miller removes all the valuable nutrients and fiber as well. The rough brown coat full of protein, oils, vitamins and fiber is removed in polishing, leaving a grain full only of starch. It is no surprise that millers do the milling and even transport free for farmers. A farmer gets grain shaped little lumps of starch called polished rice. The miller gets the rice bran, from which edible rice-bran oil is extracted. The spent bran is again nutrient rich fodder for cattle and feed for fish.

My eating of sweets or flour based products is limited to just one or two days in a week. I do eat a little more in partying and have a few drinks also on such days. I may not go to the extent of treating alcohol as Louis Pasteur did. He believed that wine is the most healthful and most hygienic of beverages. But I treat it the way I do sweets. Drinks as well as sweets, once a while and in moderation, are small pleasures of life. They need not altogether be forgone in the name of health. A feast without sweets is bland and a party without drinks, in my view, would be short and the bonhomie shallow. Both sweets and alcohol are addictive by nature. Beyond a limit, they are both equally harmful to the body. While I do not have any problem with alcohol, the fight with my craving for sweets continues. That my weakness is euphemistically called a 'sweet-tooth' is no consolation for me!

Pro-biotic Food

It is by reading a book titled "I contain multitudes" by Ed Yong and learning about the work of scientists like Dr.

Tim Spector (more about Dr. Spector and his company Zoe in Chapter 15) that I realized the important role that microbes play in my health and well being. The microbes in our body, though all together weighing a few pounds, outnumber the total number of cells in our body by several folds. There are said to be more than 1000 varieties of organisms in us producing tens of thousands of chemical compounds that are essential for the body. Only about ten of the organisms are harmful and the rest are either harmless or useful. We tend to be excessively hygienic fearing the ten organisms and in the process the other 99% are also eliminated. Even the harmless ones also help us often by outnumbering the harmful organisms. We now know that the microbes help us to breakdown our food and digest it. They also consume many of the excess calories and pass through the gut as faeces thus preventing the excess calories being a burden to our metabolic system. The most important function the microbes play is that of keeping our immune system at a very appropriate response-ready level. This helps our body from being too sensitive and thus avoid the risk of autoimmune diseases such as irritable bowel syndrome. It is also said that the gut microbes help to reduce cholesterol and body weight. Some colon bacteria, as already mentioned in this chapter, help to digest the soluble fibre in the food and convert them in short chain amino acids that are known to be anti-inflammatory and insulin suppressing.

I learnt a very convenient and easy way to keep my gut flora regularly replenished. I thoroughly mix one or two table spoons of curd and cooked grains, dilute the mix and keep it overnight for eating the next day. The several varieties of Lactobacilli in the curd that are self limited due to curdling multiply again with dilution and addition of cooked millet or rice. What I have the next day is pro-biotic rice that I hope keeps me healthy.

Soft is Hard and Hard is Easy

Whatever you eat has a serious impact on your pancreas and liver. If you eat something soft and easily digestible such as white bread or even 'healthful' brown bread or any food item and snack made of flour and sugar, your body receives a quick supply of glucose in to the blood stream. Bread and the flour based stuffs - mostly carbohydrate based - are processed several times before we eat. In the first step grain is made into finely ground flour and most of the useful fiber is removed. In the second stage it is fermented, in which the yeast digests the food for us. The third step is baking the fermented starch. The fourth step takes the bread slices to the toaster. All these steps make the work of your stomach very easy. So easy that it hardly has any work to do!

Soon after consumption of repeatedly processed food, as already discussed in Chapter 9 on hunger mechanism, the blood stream has a glut of glucose. The body cannot utilize so much glucose so soon. Pancreas and Liver start working frantically to their full capacity to regulate the excessive glucose. In doing so they over shoot their job and bring down the glucose level to lower than the minimum required level. The lower glucose levels activate the hunger mechanism. You are very soon hungry. And you eat again! The process is repeated. This food habit of yours results in:

1. Excessive sugars converting in to fat, causing overweight condition and in many cases obesity too.

2. Pancreas and liver getting, due to repeated abuse, tired too soon in life. Pancreas cannot produce enough insulin. You become diabetic.

3. Body tissues becoming insulin resistant because of exposure to too much sugar and too much insulin. They need more insulin for normal metabolic functions. High insulin content in the blood makes the tissues a little more insulin resistant. A vicious cycle is created. This is another reason for diabetes being set in.

It is measured and recorded that bread has a higher Glycemic Index (GI) than table sugar. GI is a relative index, taking pure glucose as 100, for the total rise in sugar level in the blood after the particular carbohydrate food is taken in. The foods that easily breakdown-processed, over cooked or fermented have a high GI. Most natural foods have low GI. High GI foods are advised for those who are sick or convalescing. I used to get milk with bread from the town bakery every time I fell sick during my childhood!

GI of some food products as made available in different web sites is given in the following table for easy reference:

Classification	Range of GI	Examples
High GI	70 or more	Glucose, polished or white rice, white bread, whole wheat bread, corn flakes, most breakfast cereals, water melon, dates, potato
Medium GI	56-69	Table sugar, pita bread, pasta, noodles, basmati rice, unpeeled potato, banana, dry fruits, ice cream, grape juice
Low GI	55 or less	Vegetables, most fruits, lentils, seeds, all nuts, unpolished whole grains, mushrooms, milk, yogurt

Now, on the other hand if you eat whole grain - not bread made of whole grain, but grains intact - it is quite easy for the pancreas. Your stomach has to work hard. It takes longer to digest food. Glucose is slowly released in to the blood stream. Most of it gets utilized by the body for the activities of daily life as and when it reaches the blood. Liver and Pancreas have moderate work to do. They remain healthy and last long. You do not feel hungry often as there is a slow and steady supply of glucose to the body.

A very important point to remember is that GI only indicates what type of carbohydrate food we should give preference to. The quantity of carbohydrate food we take in is an equally, if not more, important determinant in management of body weight and health. Eating unlimited low GI food cannot in any way be healthful. Ultimately it is the calorie count and quality of calories that decides your body fat levels. Another index called Glycemic Load (GL) is more important than GI. Also, GI for a food varies with the extent of processing or cooking or level of ripening. More processed or cooked or ripened food product will have higher GI.

Sugar (sucrose) has a lower GI than bread. But it does not make sugar a better food than bread. It is in fact considered as a poison by many. This is because of the reason that only one of the two components of sugar, glucose is measured in GI. The other component, fructose, which is more harmful, is not at all taken into consideration. Fructose is proven to increase fat levels in blood and increase liver and visceral fat.

One more point to remember is that if taking in of a high GI food cannot be avoided, adding a low GI food to high GI stuff would make it an overall medium GI food. For example if there is no choice but to have only white rice, adding an equal measure of vegetable to rice would make the combination a medium GI meal.

Chapter – 13

Trends Setters

It is relevant to mention here the advice of six influential trend setters who have impacted my thinking, my health and my life and who have made difference in the lives of millions, may be billions, of people world over. They are Dr. Robert Lustig, *Sadhguru Jaggi Vasudev*, Dr. *Manthena Satyanarayana Raju*, Dr. William Davis, Dr. *Khader Vali* and Dr. David Sinclair. They draw revolutionary conclusions about the food that is consumed by us, about life styles and view of life in general. These individuals' teachings or campaigns have influenced the food, mind and lifestyle of many across the world for good.

Dr. Robert Lustig

Dr. Robert Lustig, a paediatric neuro-endocrinologist, proves with his research, mass of evidence and convincing and unambiguous arguments that:

- Refined sugar (sucrose) and high fructose corn syrup, HFCS, are the reason for most of the health problems that we face. 74% of the processed foods sold in the US have these two sweeteners cum preservatives cum addictive substances generously added to boost sales and profits.

- To be more specific, fructose in these two products is the primary reason for insulin resistance and several other problems in the body.

- A calorie is not a calorie. All calories are not equal. A calorie in glucose molecules is fuel for life of all the cells of all the tissues in the body. Every cell in the body can metabolize glucose. Fructose, on the other hand, is a burden to the body because only the liver can process it. And the liver has limited capacity to process fructose. Eating a 100 calorie potato (all of it gets converted as glucose) is not the same as eating refined sugar of 100 calories, 50% of which is fructose. Glucose and fructose are isocaloric but not isometabolic.

- Sugar appears in packaged food hidden with one of its 56 names in the nutritional information provided on the pack. It's a clever way of the food industry to hide sugar. Dr.

Lusting says that real food does not need a nutritional label!

- Fructose is processed by the body in exactly same way as alcohol is processed. The only difference is that the first step of sugar to ethanol in alcohol is done outside the body by yeast. The consequences of excessive alcohol consumption, fatty liver and cirrhosis are also seen in excessive fructose consumption.

- Fructose in addition to building up liver and visceral fat, also increases triglycerides and LDL in the blood, causes wrinkles and aging and influences the addiction centers in the brain.

- Gluttony and sloth may lead to undesirable obesity. But more dangerous is TOFI, thin outside - fat inside condition of excessive visceral fat and liver fat caused by sugar consumption.

- Dr. Lustig argues forcefully that sugar has clear causative effect on obesity, type-2 diabetes and fatty liver disease and tooth decay. It has correlation for cancer and dementia too.

- He prescribes a mantra for good health in two precepts and six words: Protect the Liver and Feed the Gut. Protect the liver from the onslaught of sugar, fructose, processed foods, branched chain amino acids, trans-fats, toxins and alcohol. Feed the gut with more fibre by regularly consuming more real food – grains, seeds, nuts, vegetables and fruits.

- Dr. Lustig is not against fruits in spite of their fructose content. Fibre in the fruit is valuable. The quantum of fructose itself is very less in fruits. Whatever fructose is there in the fruit is effectively and mostly prevented by the barrier of a 'fishnet' formed by insoluble fibre and the holes in the net blocked by soluble fibre. Most of the sugar in the fruit is consumed by the gut bacteria. A juice made from fruit, on the other hand, is not healthy for the reason that the roughage of insoluble fibre is discarded in juice-making, resulting in the loss of the advantage of the barrier it creates. The fructose in the fruit is liquefied and freed for quick absorption by the intestines.

- He advises the youth to know the difference between happiness and pleasure and work towards a life of happiness. Pleasure is dopamine driven and is always short-lived. The sources of dopamine are substance like sugar, alcohol, drugs and gadgets or habits or behaviors like gambling, shopping, gaming and pornography. Happiness, on the other hand, is long lasting and is a consequence of serotonin which can be generated by good physical activity, healthy food, kind and generous heart and healthy real relationships, not virtual!

And how about the universally cherished - all time favourite of all the people - dessert? "I am for dessert", avers Dr.Lustig, "but not at every breakfast, lunch and dinner". The liver does have the capacity to process an occasional treat, not an onslaught of sugar and unhealthy fat at every meal. The body can withstand a dessert of the week-end feasting.

Dr. Lustig's YouTube talks are seen by tens of millions all over the world and his popular books, *Fat Chance*, *The Hacking of the American Mind* and the latest one, *Metabolical* are widely read. His passion to save the people from the onslaught of sugar and processed food, if he succeeds, is likely to affect the American Food Industry adversely. But he contends that what the Food Industry makes as profits is just a third of what American Economy incurs on the diseases caused by sugar and processed food.

What happens in America today generally happens in the rest of the world tomorrow. Packaged-processed foods and sodas which are sold even in the remote villages of India are likely to cause devastating long-term health issues on the populations already suffering from mal-nutrition and stunted growth. Diabetes which was rare in rural India has become quite common today. It is high time everybody got Dr.Lustig's message!

Sadhguru Jaggi Vasudev:

Sadhguru Jaggi Vasudev is a mystique, yogi and spiritual guru, social worker and environmentalist running his Isha Foundation at Coimbatore, Tamil Nadu, South India and McMinnville, Tennessee, USA. His basic teaching of life is that if an individual learns to be always joyful he or she would naturally be good to the fellow human beings, animals, plants and the environment. The identity of such an individual would never be limited by narrow boundaries of religion, colour or nationality. His identity is universal. "*Aham Bramhasmi",* he quotes a Sanskrit expression. He debunks the myth of Heaven and teasingly tells anyone who hopes to go to Heaven to go instantly, then and there. He is firm in his opinion that the idea of attaining Heaven, which was propagated by many religions, had made millions of fanatics to commit heinous crimes on humanity. His favourite joke is that of a Sunday School teacher questioning a class of little children, "What do you have to do to go to Heaven?" A few children speak about service in the church and helping the needy. But a little Tom from back bench shouts, "You have got to die first!"

Sadhguru is also for conceding "I do not know" for all things that we don't know instead of simply believing in something and taking positions. He advocates that by admitting ignorance we open up an immense possibility of knowing many things. Also, there is joy in being curious and a lot of thrill in exploration.

Sadhguru emphasizes that human body is the most sophisticated gadget on this planet and that it is a chemical factory that has a big product list. If you can manage the chemical factory well you can transform yourself to be a healthy and joyful being. The route that he suggests for good management of the chemical factory is Yoga. His trade mark course "Inner Engineering" which is a mix of a few *yogasanams, pranayamam* and *dhyanam* (meditation) is attended by millions all over the world. He argues forcefully that human body is designed by nature for vegetarian food. If one is particular about eating a protein source other than vegetarian food, he suggests that we choose from a group which is far from humans in evolutionary chart, such as fish. He is for regular fasting and says that fasting keeps the metabolic process active and also starves the cancer cells which are always there lurking in the body.

Sadhguru is of the opinion that pleasure seeking alcohol and substance abuses are the most worrying problems of the world today. Such abuse takes the present generation to a level that is lower than that of the previous generation, and that is a disaster. There is meaning to life only when a generation is better than and leads a better quality life than the previous one.

Sadhguru's videos are watched by millions across the world. He organized a programme called 'Youth and Truth' where he interacted with students of all major universities in the world. He wants to catch them young and clarify any aspect of life so that this world is a happier and better place to live in. In these sessions he answers with ease, convincingly and with absolute clarity, all sorts of questions from his audience. His amazing clarity has to be seen to be believed!

Dr. Manthena Satyanarayana Raju:

Dr. Manthena Satyanarayana Raju is a renowned naturopathy proponent based in Andhra Pradesh, India. He teaches several life style change methods with very good results for the participants of his courses. There are several books written in *Telugu* by him. He extends the old principle "see no evil, hear no evil, speak no evil" by adding "eat no evil". The 'evil' here is processed, over-cooked and tasty food. He advocates vegetarianism.

He primarily advocates eating food as much raw as possible. He is of the opinion that the food we call raw is created and cooked by the Sun. There is no need to cook over fire again. He calls the raw food as *arkapakwalu*, literally Sun cooked and cooked food as *agnipakwalu,* fire cooked. The Sun infuses life into matter and fire destroys it. He advises people to take at least 60% of the food in the form of vegetables, fruits, nuts and sprouts. He says that a family where least time is spent in the kitchen is a healthy family!

His favourite breakfast suggestion is sprouts of a mixture of grains and lentils. Sprouts as we all know are germinating seeds. We need to first soak whole grains overnight. The soaked grains are ready to germinate if we create favorable conditions for germination. A warm container with minimal aeration is generally ideal. Germination of grains takes place in 12-24 hours. A word of caution is necessary here. The ideal conditions for seed germination are also conducive to growth of harmful fungus and bacteria. We have trouble in store for the stomach and general health if we do not maintain hygiene. It is advisable to wash the grains and again the sprouts thoroughly and repeatedly with clean water. The grain used for making sprouts is believed to be a potential source of contamination. I am personally against eating sprouts as even an occasional contamination could cause an irreparable kidney damage or life threatening infection. The harmful bacteria like E.coli and Salmonella from sprouts can linger for long in the intestines and produce harmful chemicals that damage the sensitive organs like kidneys. A tragic case of sprouts contamination with E.Coli in an organic farm in Lower Saxony, Germany affecting over 3300 people resulted in death of 37 and permanent kidney damage to 818 people in 2011.

Dr William Davis:

Dr William Davis, US based author of the book *Wheat Belly* and a cardiologist has greatly impressed me with his studies and revolutionary treatment given to his patients. Dr. William Davis's conclusion is that present day wheat is very much different from the original grain. The wheat that we eat today is devoid of all good nutrients and has nothing but starch. The agricultural scientists who developed these present day strains of wheat were so focused on high yields, high disease resistance, low water requirement and short duration factors that they totally ignored the outcome. The outcome is an easily digestible, highly addictive, fiber free and nutrient deficient high-starch grain masquerading as wheat.

Dr. William Davis also advocates whole grains other than wheat, though in moderation, as regular food and proscribes all stuffs made from starch. His strong recommendation is in favour of raw nuts, which he says you can eat as much as you want. His other unrestricted foods include full-fat cheese, meat, eggs and vegetables. His limited consumption foods are milk, butter, curd/yogurt, fruits, whole grain and legumes. And his strict no are: wheat, raisins and dried fruits, all fried food, sweets and all starches. Dr William Davis equates whole grain bread with filtered cigarettes. Smoking filter cigarettes may be marginally better than non filtered ones. You are nevertheless smoking. Similarly eating whole grain bread is as bad as eating white bread, only marginally better. The concept of 'whole grains' is misused by the food processing industry to sell products which are the very opposites of 'whole'.

Dr. William Davis observes that people who reduced fat and started eating 'healthy whole grain bread' have only gained weight, visceral fat and diabetes.

He also writes that the patients who followed his wheat free diet not only lost weight but also reported relief from acid regurgitation. Patients with diabetes stopped using medicines as their diabetes was reversed. Other reported benefits are as varied as improvement in asthma symptoms to relief from rheumatoid arthritis pain.

Dr. Khader Vali

Dr. Khader Vali is a scientist based in Mysuru, Karnataka, India. His mission is to revive the almost forgotten coarse grains or millets of India; Fox tail millet, Brown top millet, Barnyard millet, Kodo millet and Little millet. He says that millet cultivation is environment friendly because it takes just 200 litres of water to grow a kilogram of millets compared with 3000-5000 litres for rice and wheat. He also teaches a system of natural farming called *kadu krishi* or jungle farming that includes a patch of natural forest within the farm to maintain a base for farmer friendly birds and insects. The small natural forest helps to maintain an ecological balance to keep the pests at bay.

Dr. *Khader* promotes consumption of millets and prescribes different millets coupled with some plant leaf concoctions as remedy for different ailments. His point in favour of millets is that:

- Millets take longer to breakdown. They take as long as six hours against less than one hour for rice and wheat. Macronutrients are very slowly absorbed into the body.

- Millets have very high fibre content. The fibre in millets is uniquely arranged in layers, with nutrients in between layers, that facilitates slow digestion.

- The amino acid profile of millets is much better than that of cereals. The better amino acid profile helps to boost the ability of the body to fight disease.

He is against consumption of meat, eggs and milk. "Why does a hen lay eggs?" he asks his audience and then goes on to answer his own question, "Because the hen wants to have a clutch of chickens, not to feed you!"

Dr.Khader's claims of cancer cure with a prescription of millets and plant leaf concoctions are rejected by many. But he is followed and respected by many diabetics and people with chronic ailments who have benefitted from his millet prescriptions. The prescription of millets as staple food perfectly fulfils the two precepts of Dr. Robert Lustig's. Millets protect the liver as they take a long time to breakdown and do not overload the liver. The rich fibre content of millets also feeds the gut!

Dr. David Sinclair

Dr David Sinclair is an Australian born geneticist. He is a researcher in the field of aging at Harvard Medical School. His recent book '*Life Span*' with subtitle '*Why We age - and why We Don't Have To*' has created a lot of interest among all people who are conscious of health, fitness and old age. His work is considered by some to have the potential to be a breakthrough that can match the discovery of antibiotics.

Dr. Sinclair concludes that there is no single cause for aging as it has been thought so far. There are, in his own words, several 'hallmarks' in the body that lead to aging and the diseases that come with it. Some such hall marks are already identified and some are yet to be known. Basically, it is the loss of information in our bodies that causes aging. The information that he refers to is of two types. One is DNA, the damages to which have been hitherto widely believed to be the most important cause of aging. Dr. Sinclair believes that DNA is generally more intact and does not get damaged much with age. The second one is Epigenome. Epigenome are a network of chemical compounds surrounding the DNA. They regulate the DNA by determining which genes are active and which are silent in a particular cell. Epigenome changes more with age, food habits, physical activity, environment, state of mind and causes the bodily changes that lead to aging.

The information loss is comparable, as per Dr. Sinclair, to an old DVD that develops scratches there by making the undisturbed data underneath (DNA that is intact) unreadable. The quest is now to find a way to even out the scratches without disturbing the data. "To be young again", says Dr. Sinclair, "We just need to find some polish to remove the scratches."

Dr. Sinclair's opinion is that we are now getting too comfortable than we were meant to be. We were evolutionarily designed to be more often hungry, face cold or hot weather and physically struggling, most of the time. These adverse conditions turn on the body to fight back. If we exercise and skip a meal (to reduce calories as well as to stress the body with hunger) to imitate those adverse conditions we would be inducing this ancient mechanism of fighting back that protects the body from decay, disease and all the root causes of aging in an effort to survive. The best way to do fasting is to skip breakfast or dinner and reduce the feeding window resulting in fasting of over 16 hours in a day as in Intermittent Fasting. Over a period, he advises to skip lunch too so that we have just one meal a day with a feeding window of just 1-2 hours. His advice about fasting is same as that of Sadhguru Jaggi Vasudev.

In addition to exercise, exposure to heat and cold, calorie restrictions and fasting which keep the survival genes on, he is also for taking of supplements to strengthen the longevity pathways and delay aging:

- NMN – Nicotinamide Mono Nucleotide is a precursor to a compound called NAD that promotes Sirtuins in the body. Sirtuins protect the body cells from damage, repair DNA, reduce inflammations and even boost memory.

- Rapamycin which is presently used as an organ transplant rejection drug is found to inhibit a kinase enzyme called m-TOR which is known to promote undesirable cellular growth. Meat consumption is known to promote m-TOR. Rapamycin helps to control m-TOR.

- Metformin which is a very safe and widely prescribed diabetes drug is found to promote AMPK, another kinase enzyme. AMPK inhibits synthesis of fat, cholesterol and triglycerides. It also helps in uptake of fatty acid and glucose by tissues. Thus metformin helps to boost overall energy of the body.

Chapter - 14

Upkeep of My Body

Exercises for me are body maintenance activity. I try to be very regular and make it as varying as possible. Though I am aware of my age and my limitations, my aim is to have an agile body. In addition to the components of fitness – strength, stamina and flexibility – agility demands good reflexes, good balance, coordination of different body parts and speed. An agile body is lithe, can react quickly to any situation. The action is swift and perfect. Balancing can be achieved by walking on an uneven ground and trying to stand on one leg. Reflexes are improved by playing games like table tennis and coordination by exercise like skipping.

I exercise a minimum of five days a week. A typical day begins with a 30 minute meditation at home. After meditation, I do 12-15 rounds of skipping rope with *Yogasanams* (standing postures) in the rest periods. Each round consists of 2 minutes of skipping, followed by a minute of rest and a minute of one *Yoga* posture. Time taken is 50-60 minutes. Another activity I undertake in some of the days is 10-12 rounds of walk-run-walk-run high intensity interval exercise for about one hour. Each round takes my heart rate to peak zone and next few minutes of walking brings it down to fat burn zone thus helping my heart with good HIIT workout.

My next activity, if I have time, is doing a 30 minute round of other *Yogasanams* before my breakfast. I ensure that I do the *Yogasanams* at least thrice a week.

If I have access to a gym I do a 30 minute brisk walk on the treadmill with a steep incline or same period of high intensity work out on the elliptical trainer. It is followed by three 10-rep sets of dead lift, squat, lat-pull, shoulder-press and biceps-curl in the gym.

On the other hand, if I am unable to do skipping due to work and I don't have access to gym, I do three 10-rep sets of biceps-curl, lateral-rise and front-rises with dumbbells at home. And if I am travelling and cannot do skipping or weights and don't have access to a gym I go out for a long walk or at least do a double round of *Yogasanams*. It is necessary to keep alive the commitment to my body, always. Time for routine basic maintenance activity of the body should be non-negotiable for any one.

In addition to the above I walk at every available opportunity. I have set myself a daily target of 18,000 steps on my Fitbit. It is a tough target, but I try to achieve at least a few times in a month.

How often do you need to exercise in a week? How many exercise-breaks do you need? Whether it is for a seasoned fitness freak or a beginner, it is universally accepted that at least one day holiday is necessary. So if you are comfortable, you can exercise on the remaining six days. But many experts advise that every strength training exercise requires a minimum of 48 hour break for the muscles to repair themselves. This means that, strength training exercise cannot be done more than thrice a week. The usual aerobic exercise can be on all the six days or on the remaining three days, if you don't want to mix aerobic and strength training workouts.

If you are a beginner, on the other hand, you have to start with just three days a week and gradually increase the duration of exercise as well as the number of days of workout ideally over a six month period. It is only by way of gradual increase that you can sustain a workout plan. If you are in a hurry to set higher goals and speed up the schedules, your body has a ready system of 'speed breakers' to stop. You will be disappointed very soon as you will be forced to stop exercising either due to illness or an injury or a sprain.

My experience with weekly holiday for exercise is that it is not quite required to specifically declare one. Most of us have important and unavoidable work, family and other social commitments that arise unexpectedly often. While there is a pressing demand from your spouse or child or reminder from your office, or a prompt from a friend for any missed activity of daily routine, there is none for a daily workout. We will invariably and generously sacrifice our daily workout because of paucity of time. Any such missed workout is a holiday by default. If such holidays-by-default happen more often I somehow squeeze in some time for *Yogasanams*. That will at least keep my body warmed up.

But it has to be remembered that there is a risk of heart attack during or after any strenuous workout. It is an exerciser's dilemma. Strenuous exercise increases your risk of heart attack. It is also true that regular exercise reduces the overall risk of death. If you are a regular exerciser your risk of getting a heart attack is much lower than others who do not exercise at all.

Fitness and regular exercises should not make you overconfident. It is necessary to go for regular health check up and get screened for health problems. Any signs and unusual symptoms should alert you to seek the help of an emergency health care professional. Ignoring the signs like breathlessness or pain with a feeling of 'nothing can happen to a fitness freak like me' is an invitation to disaster. Fitness is good, but nothing can offer total protection.

Healthy Way of Life

It is accepted by everybody that formula for fitness is regular exercise and moderate eating. It is also agreed that fitness comprising of strength, stamina, flexibility and body weight management will naturally result in good health, self-confidence, longevity and happiness. But can everybody become fit and lead a healthy, long and happy life? It is very much possible. But unfortunately, the truth is that only a few do. 'Regular exercise' and 'moderate eating' are not so simple to follow for life. They cannot by themselves sustain for long. You have to change your attitude, modify your eating habits and cultivate a life style that is compatible with your health and fitness goals. You also have to have other daily activities which promote fitness and good health. Here are some activities and life style changes that I try to follow for my fitness and health. In addition to your core fitness exercises you have to study, think and design your own life style and activities that help you to achieve your health and fitness goals.

1. **Blood Donation**

Blood Donation for me is not an act of altruism. It is a requirement for the health of my body. I thank the Blood Bank every time I 'donate' blood. The fact that my blood may save a life is only a bonus to me. While I enable a doctor to save a life by transfusion of my blood to a needy fellow human being, I am actually infusing fresh blood in to my body, literally. Every time I give blood, my body has to work and produce fresh blood cells to replenish the loss. That will make my system active and healthy. There are also many benefits that I get by giving blood.

√ Every time I give blood I have a mini health checkup which is done free. A doctor checks my blood pressure and screens my blood for any infections. There is an option to get notified if there is any negative issue about my blood.

√ My body gets rid of any excess iron which I might have accumulated. Such accumulation is very common in men and postmenopausal women. High iron levels are linked to Cardiac Problems, Cirrhosis, Cancers and Bacterial and Viral Infections. Researchers believe now that the low rate of cardiac problems in menstruating women is mainly due to their regular loss of menstrual blood and resultant lower iron levels.

√ Regular blood donation helps me to make my blood thinner each time I give blood. My body regains the reduced volume of blood by dilution with the enhanced fluid intake that is done as advised by doctors. A thin blood is free flowing and is light on my heart and vascular system. A study in Finland reported that blood donors who gave blood once a year had 88% lesser risk of heart attacks. I give blood 3-4 times a year.

√ Some evolutionary biologists believe that human body is designed by evolution for regular loss of blood. The primitive man bled regularly due to falls, attack by wild animals or injuries in fights with other tribes. That was a way for the body to get rid of excess iron and keep the blood production system functioning. But the present safe and secure life does not allow such loss of blood. Donation is an alternative way to lose blood.

√ Every time I give blood I feel happy that I have done something good to my body and also helped somebody.

√ Each donation helps me burn about 650 Calories which is more than a day's heavy workout.

2. **Putting on Shoe and Socks**

• A mundane task could be made into a fitness activity. Every time I have to put my shoes on I squat down and tie the shoe lace. It helps to stretch my leg muscles as well as strengthen my knees. It is a daily and regular exercise.

• Similarly, while I put on the socks, I do so while standing on one leg. It helps to maintain my balancing ability. It also exercises my knees and feet as the entire weight of the body is on one leg. When I started doing this daily routine, it used to be a little awkward and a little embarrassing in the presence of others. But now I am comfortable and do it with ease. It reminds me every day that I am fit and encourages me to maintain my fitness.

- Balancing on one leg helps to improve your quality of life in later years. Balancing, as already explained in Chapter 12 on plantar fasciitis, is the preparedness to make correct movements, orientation and automatic postural adjustments of the body when required. Such preparedness comes with stamina, strength and flexibility of your body. It helps to maintain stability and steadiness in activities of daily life on varying surfaces - whether you are walking on uneven ground or bending your body to avoid hitting an object or when you are getting up from bed. Inability to balance or bad balance is the single most important reason for falls and resultant life threatening fractures in old people.

3. **Grocery Shopping Trips**

- Any unplanned trip to the neighborhood grocery store in the past used to irritate me. But I realized an opportunity in the irritant. Every trip is an additional or bonus physical activity that keeps my metabolism in the drive mode. And what is more, I welcome such trips and enjoy doing it. I also readily volunteer to fetch and carry for my family.

4. **A Spring in the Step, Gleam in the Eye, a Song in the Heart and a Smile on the Face**

- Whatever I do now, I do enthusiastically because that is the way I would be energetic. Getting up and walking with a spring in the step will help me to be lively and spirited. To be happy, confident and full of enthusiasm is the motto. I also try to enthuse all around me with a smile. A smile is contagious and a simple good morning smile can create a happy environment around me. One more habit that keeps me occupied and active is my healthy and positive curiosity for things, happenings and people around. I, of course, do take care not to cross the limits, so that I am not nosy and interfering.

5. **Walk in Rail Stations and Airports**

- My best way of spending idle time at Railway Stations, Bus Stations and Airports is walking around in the available space. I do take care to walk without in any way compromising my safety and without disturbing others. It helps me to flex my leg muscles and is a healthy way of spending idle time.

- On the other hand, while in an airplane or bus or in a train chair-car on a long journey, I always keep moving my feet so that my feet do not swell. One good way of moving legs while sitting on long journeys is to write alphabets and numbers with your feet in the air below the seats. Not moving your legs while sitting on long a journey is in fact dangerous. A potentially fatal condition called economy class syndrome can result in such cases.

- In the case of economy class syndrome, the blood does not move up from the legs due to the inactivity of the muscles. While the blood in the arteries moves due to the pumping of the heart, the blood in the veins of lower limbs moves against gravity with the movement of leg muscles. Leg muscles, as explained in Chapter 7 on Bullworker, being very large and vasculature very extensive, the quantity of blood pushed up or pumped up is quite high. It is for this reason that the legs are called second heart of the body. Hours of continuous sitting in a cramped seat without moving legs will make the blood stagnant. A stagnant blood tends to clot. The blood clots may travel through and block the small blood vessels in the brain or heart and can cause fatal strokes.

6. Standing on One leg - Working or Reading While Balancing on One Leg

- I take short walks at home or try standing on one leg while on casual long phone calls. That helps me to either move around or balance my body on one leg. Even while reading or working on a computer too I try standing for short periods on one leg. It is a good exercise for my legs, especially knees.

- If I am forced to idle, as in waiting for someone in an office I spend the time by breathing slowly and consciously. The breathing energizes me and helps me to spend the idle time without getting bored. Otherwise, idle waiting tires me. The activity gives me the benefits of *Pranayamam* and *Dhyanam*.

7. Active Involvement in Hard Part of the House Hold Work

- I try to help, whenever possible, in house hold work. I do the cleaning, if necessary, of wash rooms, wall tiles, lifting heavy things, carrying bags, cleaning the attic and such work.

8. Snacking Smart on Nuts, Fruits and Pop Corn

- Snacking is one of the most important reasons why we put on weight and end up getting used to eating junk food. We need to snack when we are hungry in between meals. But most of the snacks - donuts, muffins, cakes and the like - are made from repeat processed foods - starchy, sugary, oily and even deep fried. They are full of calories and totally devoid of fiber and desirable nutrients. Over a period I have realized that snacking should be avoided or done in a healthy way. I have now got used to snacking on raw or roasted nuts or fruits or occasionally on pop corn. Nuts are rich in fiber, essential oils and protein as well. They have a low GI. Pop corn, rich in fiber and complex carbohydrates, is better than donuts and cup cakes.

9. Serving Size

I control my eating quantity considerably by reducing my serving size. If I serve myself less in the plate, I tend to eat less. Portion control is a basic aspect of weight management.

One more care I take about my food is to compensate my feasting with subsequent controlled eating during the next few days.

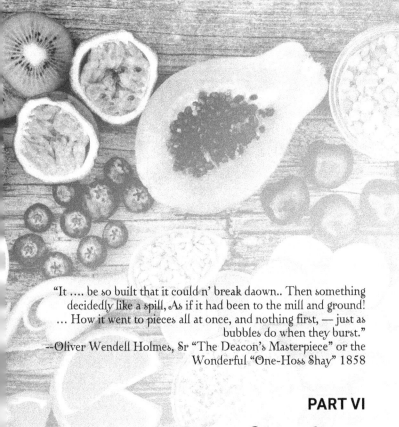

"It …. be so built that it could n' break daown.. Then something
decidedly like a spill, As if it had been to the mill and ground!
… How it went to pieces all at once, and nothing first, — just as
bubbles do when they burst."
--Oliver Wendell Holmes, Sr "The Deacon's Masterpiece" or the
Wonderful "One-Hoss Shay" 1858

PART VI

The Life Ahead

Chapter – 15

New Tools

I am now in my sixties without any fear of 'age related' issues. My focus on health and fitness continues to be more dedicated than ever. I am able to exercise better than before. I started jumping rope in my early forties. I was then doing to a maximum count of 1000. Now in my sixties, I have progressively increased the duration and can jump to a count of 5000 in one session of less than an hour. I do this activity as high intensity interval training (HIIT) exercise with brief rests in between. I have to admit, however, that my weakness for food isn't fully in control. But my food habits have improved for better. I have made several changes to my general life style. I keep searching for all new advancements and look to learn about any new trends or tools on health and fitness. There are a number of new developments in the field of health and fitness. I keep track of the developments to know and to see anything is useful to me. Given below are some interesting developments.

ZOE:

Zoe is a health science company based in the USA and UK. Zoe's rationale is that gut micro biome is the key player in the body and it can be manipulated by diet to improve overall health. They undertake to help individuals in weight loss, to improve appetite and make one feel better, increase energy levels and solve existing and potential health problems. Their service will not prescribe any medicines or supplements. It will just be changes in diet exclusively to suit your *sui generis* body and to help your extraordinarily unique micro biome to work and aid in good health.

Zoe uses a large data base with the aid of advanced soft ware, bioinformatics and machine learning programs to predict an individual's nutritional response to any food. They are said to have collected data from over one million volunteer contributors to help in their predictions. The company claims to be backed by cutting edge science with the collaboration of Massachusetts General Hospital, King's College London, Stanford Medicine and Harvard T.H. Chan School of Public Health. They do the profiling of your gut micro biome (poop test) and also collect your data through blood tests and stick-on glucometers that monitor your glucose levels every five minutes, to help them in their predictions. The company arranges for collection of regular blood and stool samples in addition to providing wearables for getting sleep and exercise data.

The scientific co-founder of the company Dr. Tim Spector says that instead of following the present system of testing blood sugar and blood fats in fasting state, Zoe does it in postprandial state because that is the state most of our lives we are in. Dr. Spector and other scientists have found to their bewilderment that though 95.5% genes are common between two different individuals, the common gut microbes between two people do not exceed 25%. In the case of identical twins whose DNA is 100% similar; the common microbes are just 33%. Due to this variance each individual is unique. An individual's response to food is also unique.

All along it was believed that diet shaped our body and our health directly. It is being proved by Dr. Spector and other scientists now that diet, a healthy diet, shapes gut micro biome also. The invisible, diversified and innumerable guests within our body are now shown to have an enormous influence on the host metabolism in a complex interplay to such an extent that a sample of an individual's gut micro biome is a better predictor of health than the individual's DNA.

Dr. Spector, surprisingly, does not recommend taking prebiotics (prebiotics are non-digestible substances like fibre that act as base as well food for microbes) and probiotic supplements unless one is taking antibiotics or suffers from gut disorders or inflammatory disorders. He compares them to vitamin supplements and advises that the way we don't need vitamin supplements when we take good diet, there is no need for these supplements when we eat a gut healthy diet. Gut healthy diet is nothing but unprocessed, diversified plant food. He suggests that we consume a minimum of 30 plant foods, consisting of vegetables, fruits, seeds, nuts and spices, in a week in addition to some fermented food. Polyphenol rich foods (brightly coloured vegetables and fruits), in addition to providing disease fighting antioxidants to the body, are also like fertilizer to the gut micro biome.

It appears to my health conscious mind that the services provided by Zoe, and any other such companies that will follow soon, will surely bring out incredible positive changes in our lives. The changes, I am sure, would not be lesser than those made by the invention of vaccines in preventing and treating diseases!

Body Volume Index:

Age, gender, body shape, ethnicity and past medical history are not taken into consideration while calculating BMI. But all these parameters are crucial in determining the risk factors for obesity and related health issues. Moreover, there is no uniformity and accuracy in measurement of height and weight of individuals; some health professionals measure the height of a person with foot wear on while others do without. Weight varies substantially with the type of clothing, foot wear and other accessories one carries on the body. An important negative indicator like abdominal fat, also known as central obesity, does not get factored in BMI. With so many shortcomings, BMI is not considered as an accurate tool any more. It is possible that an unfit individual, who is in normal BMI range could improve himself in terms of strength, stamina and flexibility and yet move to overweight category of BMI even as his fat content comes down and muscle mass increases with fitness.

Launched as a test product in 2010, Body Volume Index (BVI) is a new concept being evaluated and validated for adoption by health industry professionals. It is validated through the two-year Body Benchmark Study, a collaborative project of several healthcare research institutions in Europe and the USA. It is most likely to be launched fully very shortly. BVI takes into account the fat deposit distribution on the body of the subject by measuring even waist circumference. Unlike BMI which is calculated simply with weight and height of the subject, BVI is arrived by measuring the whole body by a 3D scanner. The scanner takes full body data - the individual has to enter a booth with just tight fitting under garments - and analyses the data to arrive at the distribution of fat on the body, obesity and health risk. It is an accurate new measurement for obesity and assessment of health risk.

The institutions involved in the validation of BVI have obtained and used body scans of over thirty thousand individuals as normative data for standardizing the index. A person's data is correlated with the normative data of the same gender, age and ethnicity and then the index is derived.

Meanwhile, a phone based app called mybvi is now available for download. The app does, for a fee, a phone-scan of the body and gives a report of your body composition based on weight distribution and body shape. It also estimates visceral fat that can indicate health risk. The app does not appear to give as good an index as the originally designed BVI that was expected with 3D scan of the body. It doesn't also seem to take ethnicity and past medical history of the individual into consideration.

23 and Me

'23andMe' which is an US based private company is first of many such companies to offer a personal genome service at an affordable price. The company sends a test kit which has to be sent back with a sample of saliva. The company analyses thousands of variable patterns in your DNA that give a clue to your different traits. Several activities and services of 23andMe are currently approved by the US Food and Drug Administration (FDA). The results and analysis are made available through the company's website and could give you an indication of your inherited traits, genealogy and ancestry: which means that the test reports give an estimate of:

1. What is your predisposition for several traits including baldness, blindness, cardiac problems, diabetes and many diseases? Such predisposition estimates can predict or warn

you to take preventive steps or prepare well in advance to face the health problems.

2. Your Genetic Health Report and Carrier Status Report which indicate any hereditary diseases that you may likely face in future.

3. Wellness Reports that can show, based on statistical models, how your DNA could influence your diet, exercise, weight and sleep.

4. Who are your genealogical DNA relatives among other people who have already got tested? You can have the pleasure of contacting people with whom you share a common ancestry. And,

5. What percentage of your genes are from which continent of the world?

Another major and probably the most useful benefit of 23andMe's work is the genetic data base the company is creating by acquiring the data from the customers as a donation. It is likely to be an invaluable asset for medical and health research. The company is also recruiting patients and is building a data bank of 'communities' with specific health conditions such as Parkinson's disease. They are also trying to profile the genome of the affected person's parents and siblings. It is said that such 'communities' are unparalleled in medical history and are invaluable in medical research. On the negative side, it is contested by some people that such data bank will create serious privacy issues.

Google Fit

There are some applications and devices that keep track of your health and fitness data. Such data keeping makes you to be constantly aware of your fitness goals. If you are constantly aware of the goals you have a better chance of attaining the goals. I use Google Fit on my mobile phone. Apple also has its own health app.

Google Fit is an app that can be downloaded free on your Android Smart Phone from Play Store. It has several features that are convenient for keeping track of your daily fitness activity. Once your basic personal data such as gender, height, weight and your goal for daily activity is entered, the application starts recording your fitness data automatically. The automatic activity recording is subject to your having the device on your person. You can, at any time, check the number of steps you have walked during the day. It even gives you a congratulatory electronic bouquet once you reach the day's target. You can check the distance travelled, time spent in walking and the calories burned too. The app shows when and where you walked or ran and for what distance at each time.

There is a provision in the app to manually feed activities or workouts like strength training or dancing or yoga for which the app will calculate and add to your calorie spends. It can also graph your activities for better viewing. The app is said to be compatible with and can be linked with other fitness devices. It will consolidate all the fitness data in to one platform if you are using other apps or devices.

But the most important lesson that I learnt is that the calorie spends that we record for the exercises are a humbling experience. We may think after a good workout that we have done well and burnt a lot of calories. But if you compare at the end of the day, the calories spent by exercises would generally be less than 25% of the total calorie spend. The remaining 75% of the day's calories are spent as 'inactive calories'. Inactive calories means the energy spent for maintaining the body. It is a fact that we spend much more for maintaining the idle body than for the activities of life. The activities of daily life and exercises need very small quantities of fuel. Eating more on the assumption that you are working out well would be a big mistake. You will be at a greater risk for obesity.

There are some drawbacks with the app that you have to keep in mind before you start using the app. The step count recorded seems to be only approximate. Its accuracy cannot be relied upon for any other purpose. The calorie count also cannot be accurate because there is no provision to enter the intensity of any exercise. Sometimes motor cycle rides or even bus rides are recorded as cycling. There is also no proper system to log your food intake and its calorific value. The app's location tracking is faulty. In spite of the drawbacks, which are mostly not relevant to health and fitness, I feel that the app is a boon to fitness conscious individuals like me. It helps me to track and be constantly aware of my fitness goals. I am sure the developers of the app will correct the defects soon and make it even more convenient to use.

Fitbit

A gift of Fitbit smart watch given by son took my fitness programme to a higher level. I learnt to use most of the functions of the smart watch very soon. There was ready normative data to check how I was doing. The most satisfying piece of data in the watch and app was that I had a cardio fitness score in the range of 50-54 (as against an excellent score of 38.7 and above for people in my age group). I was also happy that I was mostly getting a sleep score of 80-90, which is again good for any age. My curiosity made me to read everything that I could search about the gadget!

Fitness trackers like Fitbit and Apple use combination of several advanced technologies and let you know and record of many health and fitness parameters in the tracker as well as in an app in your smart phone for each day. it also keeps record of the past data.

Here are the technologies:

1. An accelerometer (3-axis) which counts the steps based on your movement. The technology can also calculate the duration of your activity, frequency and intensity too. An appropriate pattern of movement gives a more accurate results. Wearing the devise on the hand that moves is necessary.

2. An altimeter device embedded in the tracker can count floor climbing. This is done using the variation in barometric pressure and the steps taken.

3. GPS, when the tracker is connected, determines the distance run or walked. When not connected, by default, it calulates the distance based on steps. Number of steps multiplied by your stride length - which is based on your input data of height and sex - is the distance covered.

4. Medical technology called Plethysmography that can detect the minute changes in the blood volume and its flow in blood vessels under your skin by sending rapid signals and reading several parameters. This technology gives an accurate measurement of your heart rate and oxygen saturation levels in your blood.

5. Software to record, analyze, calculate, conclude and present the data as required.

6. Advanced algorithms and programming to do an analysis of your sleeping pattern, sleep timings, resting heart rate, sleeping heart rate etc.

The device is linked to your Smart phone by Bluetooth and together they provide you many features. Whether it is important to check your own fitness related data depends on your fitness level, your fitness goals, your curiosity and desire for fitness.

Is it necessary to use a smart watch like Fitbit? Let's first consider what it shows and what the uses are;

Here is what a Fitbit gives/shows:

- Steps walked

- Distance covered.

- Calories burnt.

- Active minutes with elevated heart rate.

- Real time or live heart rate and resting heart rate.

- Sleep data - hours of sleep, share of deep sleep, light sleep, REM sleep and 'awake in bed' time, comparison with bench mark sleep data for your age, 30 days average data (These are shown in bar diagram for easy glance), sleeping heart rate with graphical representation for full night view of heart rate, similar graph for oxygen variation in sleep hours and remarks about your day's sleep score.

- Tracking of weekly exercise goals.

- Hourly reminder to complete a minimum of 250 steps (for up to 14 hours in a day) and a congratulatory bouquet on successful completion at the end of the day.

- Provision to input your weight loss target and its weekly progress.

- It gives your cardio fitness score based on your exercise data. The score which is equivalent of VO2 Max in medical language indicates the ability of your system to utilize oxygen during exercise. Your score, ranging from poor to excellent in a 6-step scale, is also compared with the range for men or women of your age.

- It also analyzes your exercise session and shows how your heart performed in different ranges or zones - peak zone, cardio zone, fat burn zone and below zones.

- It gives you several options to change or set your heart rate zones, active zone minutes, active hours, step count target, calories burnt target and sleep hours.

• You get a weekly mail indicating how you performed in various parameters compared with previous week.

• You can also get an analysis of sleep data for a deeper understanding of your sleep or for any medical purpose.

Here are the several benefits of using a fitness tracker:

1. Wearing a fitness tracker is a constant reminder that you have to exercise.

2. It gives you data of your activities that can prompt you to achieve more. They encourage you by rewarding you with congratulatory messages for various landmarks in exercises that you achieve.

3. The very fact that you invested in a tracker makes it obligatory for you to put it to good use.

4. Based on parameters like heart rate or sleep score or oxygen saturation levels, and if necessary, you can seek timely medical help.

5. Some recent news reports indicate that trackers that have ECG monitoring have saved lives of people because of timely intervention by

doctors with the alarm warnings by fitness trackers.

6. My Fitbit helped me to get alerted and take precautionary treatment for Covid-19. My sleeping heart rate and oxygen variation during one night in August 2020 showed some abnormalities though I had no symptoms at all. The precautions helped me to get normal very soon. I got checked for antibodies after a month and found out that I had antibodies indicating that I was affected by Covid-19!

I don't have any doubt about the usefulness of fitness smart watches and I am certain that they do help us in getting fit!

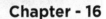

Chapter - 16

Active Life

My firm belief is that having knowledge of health and fitness, exercising or following a healthy way of life or having the most modern gadgets and tools will certainly help in your health and fitness. But none of them will be equal to a healthy attitude, a fulfilling activity and an enthusiastic mind. A life without enthusiasm and enthusiastic work cannot sustain your all other efforts. A great American Civil Rights Leader very aptly said that if a man had not found something worth dying for, he was not fit to live.

It is always necessary to have on hand an activity for which you are passionate and ever ready to sacrifice your time and energy. It should be an activity that should give reason for you to look forward to something when you wake up from sleep. It should make you move around and work the whole day. In fact even those who have normal and not a very exciting office work to attend - a work that makes them get up, get ready and get moving - would be healthier than those who have nothing to do.

I cite my experience in bank with pensioners to justify my comments. Whenever a just retired government official of sixty came to the bank to present his first pension-papers I would always wonder if he were old enough to be sixty. Most of the people looked much younger than their age. The same pensioner who came back two years later to present his annual 'not-employed' and 'life certificate', if keenly observed, would look much older than his age. Once retired and idle at home he ages very fast and looks older. He is also prone to diseases as well as depression. Just as an idle man's mind is a devil's work shop, an idle man's body is a playground for harmful germs and cancerous elements from within. Idle time leads to disuse and degeneration of the body.

On the other hand, people who have a larger purpose in life or consumed with higher objectives and lead a meaningful life never get tired and never retire. The life of a former Indian Prime Minister (PM) is an example of how an old man rose to do well a job that was thrust upon him. He was active like a young man when the responsibility of serving and saving his country fell on him. PV Narasimha Rao (PVN) took charge as Prime Minister of India at the age of 70 when India was facing bankruptcy, was about to default on sovereign payments and was facing unprecedented loss of international image. Added to his woes was the fact that he was made to head a minority government with several minor parties with divergent ideologies and some unscrupulous and highly demanding leaders. PVN, before becoming PM, was an about to retire politician. He was known as a faithful and dependable trouble shooter for the first political family of India. A Union Cabinet Minister several times, he was known as a timid old man. The only positive quality for which he was admired was his scholarship. He was a polyglot who knew 17 languages. He was chosen as the PM because he was faithful to the family that controlled the party, not considered a threat to their hold on the party and had the required Machiavellian skills to mobilize Members of Parliament (MPs) and run a minority government. Though he was known as a dull and lack-lustre politician, the quality that brought him notoriety was his slow decision making style. It was said that he would very quickly 'decide' not to take a decision on any issue at hand, how important it might be!

But the Prime Minister-ship and the responsibility of saving his country from the impending economic collapse transformed PVN in to a bundle of dynamism. Employing an economist as a Finance Minister, PVN oversaw the economic transformation of India. He was particularly known for dismantling the old industrial licensing system that was breeding corruption and driving away entrepreneurs. He took very bold and quick decisions that were unthinkable even to the so called decisive and bold Prime Ministers who had clear electoral mandate and 2/3 majority in the Parliament. He is aptly referred to as the "Father of Indian Economic Reforms". He saved Indian economy by attracting foreign investments which increased forty fold in his term of five years. He also increased defence spending that helped India face its hostile neighbours. He even boldly allowed opening of an Israeli embassy in India, in spite of the threats of backlash from Israel's adversaries.

Another small incident that showed how dynamic PVN was as PM was a reported story of his gate-crashing into a wedding. The son of a senior bureaucrat in his office was getting married to the daughter of another in the same office. The officers did not invite PVN with the intention of not troubling the 'tired old man' with his ever busy work schedules. PVN happened to learn about the wedding on the very day and just attended the ceremony uninvited with his inimitable attitude; you may not have a mind to invite, but I have the heart to bless. It is interesting to know that the groom of the wedding rose to head the top most software company of the world.

After his tenure as PM, PVN lived for a decade more as a satisfied man and wrote his autobiography.

Story of Tithonus

Many people, unfortunately, do not get any triggers for instilling a drive for fulfilling activity and an enthusiastic mind. They do not care to focus on anything other than their career and money during their prime years. They are so busy with worrying about career and business growth and savings for the retirement that they totally forget the present. They do not cultivate any taste for an absorbing hobby or have a mind to involve in a meaningful activity like service to the needy or do not have any zeal for a good cause. By the time they 'happily' retire they have a comfortable bank balance with an uncomfortable body. They are not in a position to have an engaging activity. Their only focus during retirement is getting treatment for the many health issues that they already have. It is clear that most of the people don't age well.

It appears that every retired person is dependent on the health care system for one or more problems. Added to this burden, our present health care system of attending to every problem as an isolated issue, as and when it arises, makes one like an old, poorly maintained car. An old car that is not properly serviced on a regular basis right from the beginning can't be a good car. If we merely attend to repairs as and when a problem arises we end up very soon with a shaky, rickety and undependable car. Such repairs, no doubt extend the life of the car. But it is a car that breaks down often and is not dependable. Nobody would be comfortable with such a car. In the same way many families are not comfortable with their aged parents.

The life of many old people is comparable to that of Tithonus in Greek mythology. Tithonus is the son of King Laomedon of Troy by a water nymph. He is a handsome young man when he is taken by Eos as her lover. He is proud of being loved by Eos who is a Goddess. Eos loves him so much that she wants him forever. She wants him to be immortal just the way she is and asks the King of Gods, Zeus to give a gift of immortality to Tithonus. Though a normal human being, Tithonus becomes immortal with the gift of Zeus. Eos and Tithonus thus lead a happy life.

But in the normal course of life, like any other human being Tithonus starts getting old. They realize then that they have sought immortality, but not eternal youth for Tithonus. God has granted whatever only was asked for. Thus, Tithonus grows old, becomes increasingly senile and withers away, but eternally living. He keeps praying to Almighty to grant him death and peace.

It appears that we wished for and got longevity gifted. But just the way Tithonus forgot to ask for eternal youth with immortality, we neglected to seek good health together with longevity. The developments in science, technology and medicine coupled with economic prosperity have given us the boon of lower mortality and longevity. But such a boon came packaged together with higher morbidity too. Many old people lead a miserable life of Tithonus. They regret living so long because their life is painful and wretched. Many of them feel that they are a burden to their children. Children in turn, struggling as they are with ever raising living costs or lack of time or unwillingness of their spouses and children to support, also feel the burden.

But is there a way to be healthy as long as we live and be not a burden to any one? Can we remain independent throughout? Or at least, can we minimize dependency? Some scientists believe that it is possible! They believe that one need not lead a painful and dependent life in old age. A life of impaired ability to see, hear or move and a life of declined cognitive ability can altogether be avoided. An old person can minimize or altogether avoid being under nursing care!

Story of One Hoss Shay

In American poet, Oliver Wendell Holmes, Sr's poem "The Deacon's Masterpiece" (Also called "The Wonderful One-Hoss Shay") a fictional Deacon crafts a wonderful one-hoss shay, a simple cart pulled by one horse. It is built in such a skillful way that it cannot break down. The cart is constructed from the very best of materials so that there are no weak spots. Each part is as strong as every other part. The cart endures and works perfectly for a hundred years and then all at once breaks in to heap of umpteen pieces - "went to pieces all at once and nothing first - just as bubbles do when they burst." It is irreparable. There is nothing like a breakdown time. It works well all along and at the end of its life collapses all of a sudden and meets its end. No repairs and revival are possible.

If only humans could have such a 'no-breakdown' life and such a sudden end! Or could we aim for almost such life and such end?

Fortunately, it is now felt by many scientists and doctors that postponement of all age related illnesses with proper nutrition, good fitness and a positive attitude will help to compress the morbidity and enhance quality of life. Such life will result in fewer days as dependents. It has been even observed that if onset of the first age related illness is delayed as much as possible, the period of age related illness is shortened and death is often sudden, just as in the story of one hoss-shay. If sufficiently postponed, some ailments like cancer, diabetes, hypertension and cardiac disease can altogether be prevented during the life time. It would be a painless and peaceful death after the natural life span.

Our aim, however, need not be to prolong life beyond normal years. It should only be for a qualitative improvement of the natural life; a full life of youthfulness and vitality. Such life and end means that one will be less dependent on others. There would not be much of hospitalization or nursing. The period of disability would be shorter. It also means less trouble to the children because their responsibility of looking after the ailing parents is less. In terms of self respect of the aged it would be an invaluable advantage.

And for the Economy it would also mean less expenditure on health care. The loss of man hours due to nursing and care by the attendants would also come down. Healthy old people are useful caretakers of the family and are great companions to small grand children. Their presence and care is even more desirable if both the parents are working because it is convenient and beneficial to the children and reassuring to the parents. A child in the loving care of grandparents is safer, healthier and happier than in the care of a crèche!

Chapter - 17

My Exercises

Walking

Walking is the best of all exercises. Human body is naturally designed for walking. It is universal and can be done by people of all ages at any time of day or night and practically everywhere. It is an exercise by default for anyone. Walking is also a good relaxing pastime. Some people walk to relax, some to enjoy the outdoor air and nature. Some spend their leisure in walking. Some have the habit of having pre-prandial or postprandial walks. But walking as an exercise could be effective and give substantial health benefit only if it is faster than 4kmph (2.5mph). If you walk slowly, the benefits are minimal, but are still better than being idle. Walking, however slow it might be, makes you carry your own weight around.

If walking for exercise is undertaken, it should be done with a purpose in mind; purpose of attaining fitness. One should walk firmly and with concentration so that he gets the full benefit of exercise. I don't advise listening to music while walking for exercise because it affects concentration and reduces pace. A walk which is done on purpose and with concentration gives you three benefits:

1. Physical Exercise for the body as whole,

2. Meditation for the mind,

3. Release of mood enhancing chemicals.

Walking Faster:

Walking should be done faster as your exercise program progresses. Unless you increase the speed you will not get a proper exercise for your heart, lungs, circulatory system, legs and the rest of the body. If you maintain the same speed and same style for months and years, your fitness will reach a plateau. Increase in speed gives a fresh challenge to the body and makes it gear up for higher performance. You can also alternate between moderate speed and high speed walks during the exercise session for better results. Alternating high and moderate intensity walking is an effective way of weight reduction.

Walking on an incline:

You can also walk on steep roads to challenge your heart and lungs. If it is on a treadmill you can increase the incline and get the high resistance. A steep road or an incline on the treadmill involve carrying your body weight to a higher level. Carrying a weight to a higher level demands more blood supply with more oxygen from the system. More demand means that the heart and lungs have to work more and work harder. That gives higher exercise for cardiovascular and breathing system.

Walking on Different Terrains:

Changing the surface of walking, after reaching a level of fitness, gives the body the differential stress it needs to exercise large groups of muscles, tendons, ligaments and joints. Walking on uneven surfaces helps to improve balance (as explained in Chapter 12 under 'Unusual Pain in My Foot') that is needed in times of exigencies. If your balance is good you can prevent falls and resultant injuries and fractures.

Different Styles of Walking:

Changing the style of walking involves different muscle groups and puts different type of stress on the body.

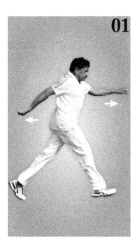

1. A brisk walk with full swing of the arms as shown Image-1 will give an excellent workout to most parts of the body. This walk gives full thrust of arms as well legs to move the body forward. The stride is quite long and arms fully extended. For every step of the walk, the foot strikes the ground with the heel and rolls to the toes and then takes off. Though the main thrust forward is achieved by pressing the forefoot on the ground it is called rare-foot strike because the heel strikes the ground first.

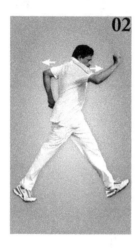

2. Another variant of the brisk walk is as shown in the Image-2. In this walk the arms are bent at the elbows. The fore arms are parallel to the ground. The shoulders give full thrust. The stride is long. In this walk both heel and ball of the foot strike the ground at the same time. It is called mid-foot strike.

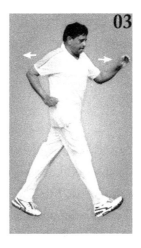

3.   Image-3 shows another style. Here the thrust is given by the waist along with shoulders. The stride is not long. The waist twists and pushes the body forward. Though both heel and ball of the foot strike the ground, the pressure is more on the ball of the foot. It is a forefoot strike. This type of walk may look funny as done by the race walkers, but is a demanding exercise.

There is no problem with rare-foot strike if it is a normal walk and if the foot rolls to the toes. But if you walk with heavy steps as in stomping or run with rare-foot strike there is a possibility of injury as the heel is not a good shock-absorber.

It is reported in a 2012 study of Harvard University Runners that people who had a habit of striking the ground with heel had twice the risk of repetitive stress injuries when compared with those who had forefoot strike. In forefoot strike the toes and ball of the foot absorb the shock of the body weight hitting the ground. It is for this reason that skipping rope is a safer exercise than running.

Running

I had given up the thought of running two decades ago when I suffered knee problems. But I was comfortable skipping and also brisk walking. My walking was quite good and could even take my heart rate to peak levels. It was at this juncture that I happened to read a book by Christopher McDougall, *Born to Run.* The book transformed me from a reluctant to an enthusiastic runner, in a very small way though. The author recites an aphorism attributed to Roger Bannister who was the first man to break four-minute mile in running. "Every morning in Africa, a gazelle wakes up," says the quote. "It knows it must outrun the fastest lion or it will be killed. Every morning in Africa, a lion wakes up. It knows it must run faster than the slowest gazelle, or it will starve. It doesn't matter whether you're a lion or a gazelle – when the sun comes, you'd better be running." The author also quotes an eccentric American runner known as Dipsea Demon, *"You don't stop running because you get old, you get old because you stop running"*!

Christopher McDougall's conclusion based on his own study and experience and authentic research by scientists like Professor Dennis Bramble and Dr. David Carrier at University of Utah and Dr. Daniel Lieberman at Harvard is that human body is specifically designed for running, more specifically, long distance endurance running. The researchers are of the opinion that Homo sapiens's running advantage helped him to have an edge over his fellow hominid, Homo erectus - who otherwise had a superior body, better hunting skills and a larger brain - in the evolutionary race. The researchers have found 26 morphological and anatomical resources in the body that helped Homo sapiens to run. Some of these advantages are:

- Foot with an arch that cushions the impact of running. The foot together with its arch is a complex and marvelous piece of engineering and architecture consisting of 26 bones, 30 joints, and more than 100 muscles, tendons and ligaments. The short and straight toes are also supportive of running.

- Achilles tendon that connects calf muscles to the heel is prominent in humans. The tendon works like spring and helps to give the jump to run. It isn't used at all in walking.

- The gluteus maximus or butt which is quite big and unique to humans is there to prevent falling forward while running. In fact the butt muscles do not get tightened when we walk. They do when we run!

- Sweating Mechanism that can cool the body on the go, unlike other animals which have to stop and pant with a tongue-out open mouth to cool off the body.

- Nuchal ligament in the neck connecting the head to the trunk to keep the head stable in the same way as other running animals like horses and dogs. Walking creatures like pigs and chimpanzees don't have the ligament.

- Very efficient diaphragm to aid in breathing.

- A very efficient balancing mechanism in the ear to help to keep the bipedal human body steady

A very relevant finding by researchers that emphasizes running by even senior citizens is performance peaking and decline with age. Starting at age 19 a runner's performance peaks in a span of 8 years at 27. The decline in performance, astoundingly, spans 37 years to reach the level of 19 at age 64. It indicates that even a 60 year old can compete in running with a young man of one-third his age!

Christopher McDougall's one more interesting recommendation is that we run minimally shod, shod just enough to safeguard your soles from sharp objects. Thin soled inexpensive shoes can serve the purpose. His reasoning based on several studies by scientists like Dr.

Daniel Lieberman is that wearing cushioned shoes block the body from getting the necessary sensory input to prepare the feet, heels and knees for the impact. A foot wear with the least cushioning feeds the body with the right input leading to adequate preparation and prevents injuries. It seems that we wasted lot of money in buying expensive shoes all these years!

Some well trained athletes who reach a high level of exercise experience a feeling called 'runner's high'. It is a feeling of being on the top of the world because of elevated state of the senses. It is a feeling of accomplishment and an exercise induced euphoria. It is explained by scientists and doctors that the euphoric feeling is a result of release by the body of endorphins, our own self produced opiates, to combat physical stress and pain. Other similar chemicals like nor-epinephrine, dopamine, and serotonin are also produced by the body during higher levels of exercises. These compounds also help to reduce inflammation and improve overall mental well being.

Skipping

Skipping Rope or Jump Rope is the simplest and most inexpensive exercise. The rope helps to gain endurance, foot work, coordination, swiftness of movements and agility. It exercises both the lower and upper body and improves cardiovascular fitness. The jumping rope tones a number of muscles of the body. Though it is wrongly considered by some as just a school girls' fun activity, its usefulness can be appreciated by the fact that it is the basic conditioning exercise for boxers.

Though jumping the rope is very simple, it needs time to get used to. Tripping on the rope is the most common obstacle for beginners. It is necessary to practice and become proficient in the use of the rope. It demands coordination of foot and arm movements and balance of the whole body. If you want to go straight to endurance level exercise with the rope, you will be frustrated. It is best to begin doing ten-second rounds of jumping with brief intervals of rest and progressively increase the duration of skipping time till you are able to do 2-3 minute rounds at one go. Thereafter you can do number of such rounds of jumping that suit your endurance level with appropriate rest intervals in between.

Skipping the rope primarily exercise the calf muscles. But along with it you also exercise deltoids, pectorals, abdominal muscles, quadriceps, and hamstrings. The muscles and joints of the feet, knee joints, hips, spinal cord and even the neck receive the repeat pounding and get hardened too. In the process the bones of the body also get strengthened. More over since the body jumps off the ground, a number of muscle groups called the 'jumping chain' work to maintain the balance and keep the body stable. Though the jump rope exercise scores high on benefits, it is a lower impact activity than running or jogging for the knees as the body lands on the toes and balls of the feet and not on the heels. Toes are natural shock absorbers of the body.

You can also imitate the jumping rope without the rope. You have to simultaneously jump and move your hands as if you are turning the rope. There is no botheration of tripping. It may not give you the benefit of hand-leg movement coordination, but gives you all the other benefits of skipping. One more advantage with imitating the rope is that you can extend the arms to different levels so that the deltoids, pectorals and muscles of the arms are exercised with different intensity.

If you advance your jump rope activity, there are number of variants to make it tougher and more challenging.

Running in place is a variant of jump rope where you skip and run remaining stationary at one place.

Double under is another variant where you jump high enough and spin the rope fast enough to slip the rope twice under the feet in one jump.

Crisscross pattern is still more difficult and needs high level of coordination. While doing the normal skip, you cross the arms so that a loop of the rope is formed in front of you. You jump through the loop and open the loop by uncrossing the arms for the next skip. You repeat the jump.

Strength Training

Strength is the basic requirement of life. Without strength you cannot lead a normal life. When you are strong you have more muscle, less fat. Your bones, joints, ligaments and tendons are also strong. You can move faster, work longer or play better. You have a healthy heart and superior fitness. When you have more muscle and less fat, your lipid profile is good with higher levels of HDL (Good Cholesterol). With all this comes improved metabolism that helps you among other things, to keep your body weight in check and to recover faster from illness or injury. Strength and good muscle mass, as explained in Chapter 6 discussing organ reserve, help you through old age with better health, better balance and quality life.

It is very well known that we need to build muscle to increase strength. But building muscle is not a simple and ready to do process. Your body has to build muscles on its own. The body builds muscle only when there is a need for the tissue. There should also be resources available for building the muscle. Your job is to create that need as well as provide the resources required. The need has to be created in the form of a task. The task is such that it places a demand on the specific muscles to work to such an extent that it is extremely difficult for the existing muscle to perform with the available muscle mass. Such task can be in the form of a strength training exercise or actual physically demanding work.

When the task is demanding enough, the need for more muscle is created. The need is actually a trauma for the muscle fibers and it acts as a stimulus for the body to build bigger and stronger muscles. The process is called hypertrophy. The loss of muscle mass with age and disuse is known as sacropenia.

There are a number of exercises that can be done to increase muscle mass and strength. It is advisable to initially seek the help of a trainer to start the strength training and to know different exercises that can be done with free weights, bar bells and gym equipment. Once you learn the technique of doing you can choose the ones which are most suitable to you and workout regularly. You have to target a few muscles each time and practice.

It helps to be familiar with some of the terms used in strength training. The lifting of a weight up at one time is called rep or repetition. 5 or 10 or 20 reps done without a break make a set. For example if you lift a dumbbell up 20 times continuously, it becomes one set of 20 reps. You need to take a break before your next set. Generally higher weights are done with less number of reps and lighter weights with higher number of reps. High weight with fewer reps(less than 5) increase muscle mass but do not help much in building endurance. Workout with lighter weights and more (12-20) reps tones the muscles and helps build endurance but does not increase the muscle mass. A workout in between, with medium weights and 6-12 reps is good for both muscle building and endurance.

Squat is a whole body exercise. When you squat down and get up, the lower body muscles push the body up. Dead lift on the other hand does both push and pull functions of the body. The lower body muscles push the body and chest and arm muscles pull the weights. Bench-press strengthens pectoral muscles. You need the help of a trainer while doing this exercise with bar bells of appropriate weight. Arm curls with dumbbells and pull-ups exercise the biceps. Dips are for the triceps. Doing the front raise or lateral raise with dumbbells exercises the shoulder muscles. The lat-pull down exercise on the gym equipment is the best exercise for your back. It strengthens the latissimus dorsi or lat muscles. It can give your body a tapered appearance with strong and big upper back muscles.

Practice of Yoga

Yogasanams: It is important to remember about all *Yogasanams*.

1. *Yogasanams* are not aerobic or strength training exercises. You have to practice at a slow pace, in a comfortable position and with a cool mind. There should not be stiffening of any muscles other than the ones involved in the posture. The sitting and lying postures are to be done on a carpet or a thin mattress.

2. But just as in the case of exercises, *Yogasanams* should also be done on an empty stomach, preferably early in the morning after your daily chores and exercises.

3. If you are unable to attain any posture fully, do not be frustrated. Stretch to the extent possible for you, without exerting yourself. Within a few days or weeks, you will easily be able to achieve the full posture comfortably. The best method to progress is to stretch as far as you can comfortably go and then stretch a little further in the final moments of the posture.

4. Practice *Yogasanams* after your workout. It relaxes the muscles.

5. *Yogasanams* help you to expel the entrapped gases from your alimentary canal either by burping or by breaking wind. They also activate the viscera, press and massage the other internal organs and improve blood circulation. Your overall mental and physical health improves.

6. My personal experience teaches me that regular practice of *Yogasanams* reduces my untimely appetite and helps me to be satisfied with less. On the other hand all other aerobic and anaerobic exercises make me to eat more.

7. There are hundreds of *asanams* in *yoga*. The 14 *asanams* described below are the asanams that I practice and are easy to follow. They stretch most parts of the body. It is not necessary to practice all every day or all at one time. An *asanam* like Supta Matsyendrasanam (Sl No.8 and Image-11) can be practiced on the bed too. It energizes you to start the day. All the standing posture asanams (Sl No. 11-14. Images-14 to 18) can be practiced when you go for a walk. If you are short of time, you can just do a few *asanams* so that you don't skip the routine altogether.

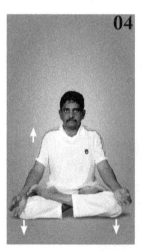

*1.   **Padmasanam** or **Lotus Pose**: (Image-4) Sit cross legged on the floor with your body erect. Keep a level head, figuratively too. Place your right foot on the left thigh and the left foot on the right. Extend and rest your arms on your knees, palms facing up. The index and thumb join together to form a ring. The other three fingers are straight and relaxed. Breathing is deep and slow. It is the most preferred posture for meditation. Once you are comfortable with *Padmasanam*, you can continue sitting in the posture for as long as you wish to and do *pranayamam* and meditation. It is a comfortable posture for reading too.

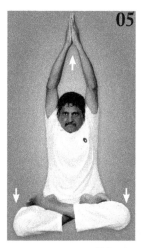

2. *Parvathasanam* or Mountain Posture: (Image-5) Assume *Padmasanam* Posture. Join your palms in front of your chest as in a '*namaste*'. Then slowly raise the arms with joined palms high over your head so that the upper arms touch the ears. Breathe in while assuming the posture. Hold your breath and remain in the posture for 8-10 seconds. Lower your arms slowly while breathing out. Repeat the asanam 4-5 times.

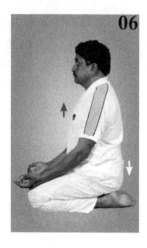

3. *Vajrasanam* **or Ankle Posture:** (Image-6) Start in kneeling position so that upper side of your feet rest on the floor and soles look up. Your body is erect and head is at correct level. Slowly sit and rest your body on your heels and rest your arms on your knees. Breathing is deep and slow as in *Padmasanam*. This *asanam* is also a meditative posture.

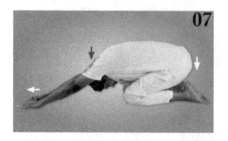

4. *Shashankasanam* **or Moon / Hare Posture:** (Image-7) Sit in *Vajrasanam*. Raise your arms above the head palms facing forward. Slowly breathe in. Bend forward with outstretched arms, while breathing out, so that the fore head and arms rest on the floor. Remain in the position without breathing in for 8-10 seconds. Come back to original position slowly breathing in. Repeat 4-5 times. If you want to prolong the posture, you can remain so with slow breathing.

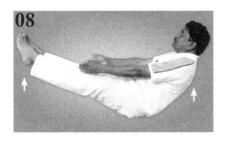

5. *Naukasanam* **or Boat Posture**: (Image-8) Lie down on your back. Raise both your legs slightly up (by 25-30 degree) and then raise your body too to the same level so that only your glutes are on the floor. Arms should be stretched to touch the knees. Breathe normally and remain in the position as long as you can. The abdominal muscles get the full contraction in the posture. Quadriceps, knees and pectorals also are stiffened. Repeat 4-5 times.

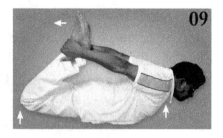

6. *Dhanurasanam* or Bow Pose: (Image-9) Lie face down on the floor. Fold the legs backwards at the knees. Extend your arms behind you and grab the ankles with your hands. Raise your head and chest simultaneously pulling the ankles with your hands so that a 'bow' is formed. Breathe in while assuming the position, hold breath while you remain in the posture for 8-10 seconds and breathe out when you slowly release your hands and come back to resting position. Repeat 4-5 times.

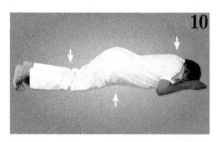

7. *Sashtanga Namaskaram* or Prostration Pose: (Image-10) Lie face down on the floor with your forearms resting by your side. Exhale and raise your abdominal region up in such way that only your feet, knees, forearms, chest and forehead touch the ground. Remain in the position for 8-10 seconds and relax while inhaling. Repeat 4-5 times.

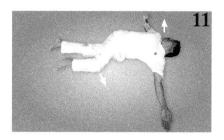

8. *Supta Matsyendrasanam*: (Image-11) Lie on your back with your arms out-stretched. Turn your head fully to the left. Bend your left knee with the sole of your foot resting on the floor and drawn close to your body. Swing the bent knee to your right in such way that it touches and rests on the floor. With both the shoulders firmly on the floor, try to fix your focus on the left palm. Breathe slowly and normally. If necessary, till you get used, you can use your right arm to press down the left knee to the floor. Complete the round with the other leg. Repeat the asanam 4-5 rounds.

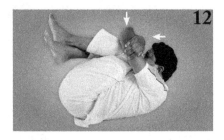

9. ***Dwipada Basthikasanam or Bipedal Antiflatus Pose:*** (Image-12) Lie on your back on the floor. Raise both your legs slowly and draw them close towards your chest by folding at the knees. Clasp the knees with both the arms and press firmly against your abdomen and chest. Remain in the position for some time with your head flat on the floor with slow breathing. Then raise your head while exhaling and try to touch the knees with your fore head. Remain in the position for 8-10 seconds and return to normal position while inhaling. Repeat 4-5 times.

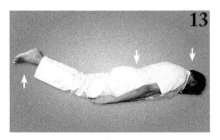

***10. Salabhasanam* or Locust Pose**: (Image-13) Lie down flat face down with your chin resting on the floor, feet together, the soles of your feet facing the ceiling and arms straight and flat on the floor by your side. Now breathe in, hold your breath, stiffen your legs and lift them up slowly. Remain in the position 8-10 seconds. Return to normal position slowly breathing out. Repeat 4-5 times. It may be difficult to do the asanam initially. You can start with trying to lift one leg each separately and practice for some days. You can then try both the legs together.

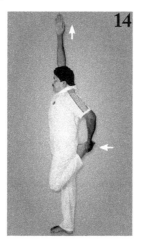

11. Santulanasana: (Image-14) Stand erect on your left leg. Fold back the right leg at knee and lift it up. Hold your foot behind you with your right hand and press the heel against your bottom. Now lift your left arm straight above your head so that it is parallel to the body and upper arm touches your left ear. Look straight ahead. Breathe in while assuming the posture. Maintain the posture holding the breath for 8-10 seconds and breathe out while coming back to normal position. You can complete one round of the asanam by standing on the right leg and repeating the process of pressing the left heel. Repeat the asanam 4-5 rounds.

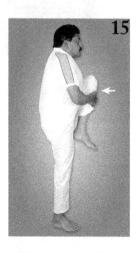

12. *Pawanamuktasanam*: (Image-15) Stand erect on your left leg looking straight ahead. Lift your right knee up in front of you and hold it with both the hands. Now press the knee tightly against the chest while breathing out. Remain in the position for 8-10 seconds and release the knee while breathing in and coming back to normal position. Complete the round by standing on right leg and pressing your left knee to the chest. Repeat 4-5 rounds.

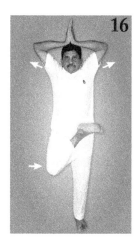 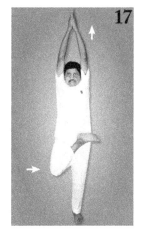

***13. Vrikshasanam* or Tree Posture**: (Images-16 and 17) Stand erect on your left leg. Lift your right foot up in front of your body, hold the heel with both the hands and place it on the top portion of your left thigh, almost on the hip. Your right knee is brought close to the left knee so that there is least pressure on the thigh where your heel is resting. Now lift your arms up and bring the palms together. Place the joined palms on the crown and stretch your elbows backwards. Breathe normally and remain in the position for 8-10 seconds. Come back to original position and complete the round by standing on right leg and by placing the left heel on the right thigh. Repeat 4-5 rounds. Another variant of the asanam is to raise your arms fully as in *Parvathasanam* and hold breath for 8-10 seconds.

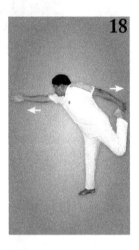

14. *Natarajasanam*: (Image-18) Stand on left leg. Slightly bend your right leg at the knee and lift it up backwards. Stretch back your right arm and hold the right foot at the toes. Now as you pull your right leg towards your body from behind, bend your body forward with your left arm extended straight and parallel to the ground. Also try to outstretch your right leg. Breathe normally and remain in the position for 8-10 seconds. Standing on the right leg and doing the asanam would be one round. Repeat 4-5 rounds.

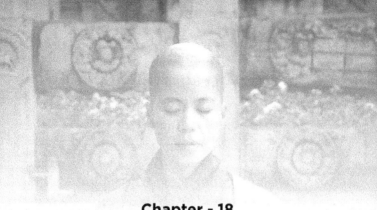

Chapter - 18

My Fitness Benefits!

Having told about by story and my fitness journey, let me summarize the benefits of fitness!

Fitness and resultant good health ensure long quality life and enable you to lead your life as per your plans. More important, it enables you to live long enough to enjoy a life of your choice, to fulfill your dreams and commitments to your loved ones and dependents.

1. Fitness keeps you in good health always and in general saves on your medical bills. It is well established that the most serious diseases affecting us today, heart disease, hypertension, diabetes and even cancer can be prevented by keeping oneself fit.

2. Fitness enhances your performance in work in two ways:

a) You have stamina to work, if required, long hours without getting drained.

b) Your efficiency improves because of your ability to concentrate better on the job.

3. Fitness improves your self-confidence and keeps you in relatively positive and happy mood all the time. This is because of higher levels in the blood of chemical compounds called endorphins, which are produced in the body when you are physically active. Confidence and positive attitude lead to good inter-personal relations, which help you to be successful in your career, family and social life. Physical exercises, Yogasanams, Pranayamam and Dhyanam are the best cures for anxiety and depression.

4. Fitness is proved to enhance sexual prowess by prolonging excitement and enhancing self-control.

5. Fitness provides immunity against many infections, diseases and even allergies. It also helps in faster recovery from illness, if any at all. Healing of wounds, injuries and cuts is much faster in fit persons.

6. When facing a dangerous situation, you are better equipped either for a fight or flight. Your

reflexes are quick and the reactions immediate in hazardous situations. Quick reflexes and appropriate swift reactions coupled with an ability to concentrate on the task on hand will greatly help, in my firm view, to be a safe driver too.

7. A fit person has better looks than an unfit one. A good body posture and proportionately built body makes one good looking. The body movements are graceful. "Fitness being the basis of beauty, nobody could have denied that his steady swings and turns in and about the flock had elements of grace." Says Thomas Hardy, describing farmer Gabriel Oak in the English classic novel, *Far from the Madding Crowd*.

8. For those who play vigorous games and participate in competitive sports, fitness helps by reducing the risk of injury. A fit individual has lesser risk of injury or spasms. Fitness training is essential for all sportspersons.

9. Food is one of the greatest pleasures of life. A fit person can continue to enjoy eating all varieties of foods without any restrictions, though moderation is required to keep the body fat and body weight in check.

10. Fitness improves sleep pattern and reduces tiredness. Your need for sleep actually comes down with fitness. You are fully refreshed with fewer hours of sleep.

11. A fit person's body is supple and agile. He can make wide range of movements comfortably.

12. If you are fit, your dependency on others, even in advanced age, is less. You can lead a dignified and independent life.

Epilogue

Civilization has brought about far reaching changes for human beings and the human body. While civilization gave him the comfort and security of community living and protection from elements and wild animals, it also made him face communicable diseases and wars with resultant disease and destruction. It provided some sort of food security in terms of division of labour, sharing of resources and also sharing of knowledge of resources. But along with that came agriculture, introducing grain cultivation. Grains, no doubt, filled hungry stomachs and mitigated hunger, but gave less protein, less variety of food and less of other nutrients to the human body.

Industrialization and mechanization further brought devastating changes to the human body. Reduction of manual labour coupled with processed food made humans fat and unfit. Globalization is taking automation to even higher levels with easy transfer of knowledge and technology. It is providing cheap and variety food easily due to economies of scale and efficiency in inter-continental logistics, and in the process, almost erasing the concept of seasons and seasonal food. Evolutionarily the human body (as well as bodies of domesticated animals too) faces strange conditions; Excess food, easy electrical and fossil fuel energy, minimum work for the body and stressful conditions for the mind.

Though the world is progressing well today in terms of wealth, science and technology, comforts and conveniences, medicine and cure of disease, there is regression in terms of disease prevention, fitness and happiness of individuals. It is well documented that more than two-thirds of the US population is either obese or over weight. Some small communities of people living in far-off islands, who depend primarily on processed, canned and frozen foods are reported to be over 80% obese. While the developing and poor countries are far behind the advanced countries in positive health, social and economic indicators, they are competing with them in obesity.

If we see the weight profile of people as recently as 1970 or 1980 and compare it with today's weight profile it can be noticed that there is substantial change. You can observe the old videos showing football or cricket matches where all the players are thin. But the present day players, who probably exercise and practice equally, if not more, look heavier. The difference seems to be in the food we take today and general slowdown in the other activities of daily life.

We use mixer grinders, blenders, dish washers and washing machines at home to save time and energy. We go to work and even for exercise on automobiles, all to save time and energy. But we expend calories by walking for an hour on an electrically operated tread mill. It is strange that the saved 'labour' is spent as 'calories' and in the process some more electric power is used to run the tread mill.

On the issue of health of people governments all over the world focus more on cure of disease. Prevention aspect is totally neglected. There used to be a Department for a subject called 'Social and Preventive Medicine' in Medical Colleges. It is now renamed as 'Community Medicine'. Even if the syllabus remains the same, the change of name suggests that the focus has shifted from 'prevention' aspect of diseases. This has to change so that students are sensitised to encourage people to be fit and to prevent disease so that the burden of the sick population on the society is less. The change could be right from primary school level so that a child grows up learning about fitness and prevention of disease.

In my view, ideally, exercising for maintaining body weight is not at all desirable. It has to be taken care of by the routine living habits. We have to cultivate the habit of doing manual work as much as possible. We need to reduce calorie intake by limiting carbohydrate consumption and altogether avoiding refined sugars, starches, processed and junk food. Exercising should be for building strength, stamina and endurance and for flexibility. And that should be achieved, as far as possible, by productive work.

It is time leaders as well as people took serious decisions to promote activities to prevent illness and improve health and fitness of everybody.

Some simple ideas are:

1. Creation of pavements for walking and tracks for cycling on every road.

2. Statutory provision of parks and walking tracks in every colony and apartment complex.

3. Giving high importance for inculcating healthy eating and activity habits in children right from elementary schools.

4. Incentivizing starting of gyms and health clubs.

5. Giving discounts for fitness in health and life insurance premium.

6. Promoting cultivation, easy supply and availability of millets and pulses at affordable prices.

7. Printing warnings on processed, fried and sweetened foods as is done for cigarettes and alcohol.

8. Introducing a system for rewarding the healthiest man and woman in each age group for every village, town and city.